Medical Radiology

Diagnostic Imaging

Series Editors

Hans-Ulrich Kauczor
Paul M. Parizel
Wilfred C. G. Peh

The book series Medical Radiology – Diagnostic Imaging provides accurate and up-to-date overviews about the latest advances in the rapidly evolving field of diagnostic imaging and interventional radiology. Each volume is conceived as a practical and clinically useful reference book and is developed under the direction of an experienced editor, who is a world-renowned specialist in the field. Book chapters are written by expert authors in the field and are richly illustrated with high quality figures, tables and graphs. Editors and authors are committed to provide detailed and coherent information in a readily accessible and easy-to-understand format, directly applicable to daily practice.

Medical Radiology – Diagnostic Imaging covers all organ systems and addresses all modern imaging techniques and image-guided treatment modalities, as well as hot topics in management, workflow, and quality and safety issues in radiology and imaging. The judicious choice of relevant topics, the careful selection of expert editors and authors, and the emphasis on providing practically useful information, contribute to the wide appeal and ongoing success of the series. The series is indexed in Scopus.

For further volumes: http://www.springer.com/series/4354

Geoiphy George Pulickal
Tiong Yong Tan · Ashish Chawla
Editors

Temporal Bone Imaging Made Easy

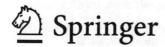

Editors
Geoiphy George Pulickal
Department of Diagnostic Radiology
Khoo Teck Puat Hospital
Singapore, Singapore

Tiong Yong Tan
Department of Radiology
Changi General Hospital
Singapore, Singapore

Ashish Chawla
University of Colorado
School of Medicine
Denver, CO, USA

ISSN 0942-5373   ISSN 2197-4187   (electronic)
Medical Radiology
ISBN 978-3-030-70637-1   ISBN 978-3-030-70635-7   (eBook)
https://doi.org/10.1007/978-3-030-70635-7

This Springer imprint is published by the registered company Springer Nature Switzerland AG
The registered company address is: Gewerbestrasse 11, 6330 Cham, Switzerland

To my wife Wern Hui, whose sacrifices for this book and my life in general cannot be measured.
To my parents George and Philomina Pulickal, who gave me more freedom and love than I ever deserved.
But most of all to my Lord, who saw fit to bless me with these people. Philippians 4:13.

Thank you.
Geoiphy George Pulickal

For my parents whose blessings, sacrifices, and inspiration keep me moving on this academic path. Thanks to my loving wife and kids for their support.

Ashish Chawla

I would like to dedicate this book to all my ENT colleagues, who through regular feedback and close working relationships over the years have greatly enhanced my journey as a head and neck radiologist. Your contributions to my own learning are immense, without which the compilation of this book would not have been possible.

Tiong Yong Tan

Preface

Throughout most of my radiology training the mere prospect of having to report a temporal bone scan used to fill me with utter dread. The anatomy was minuscule, the pathology complex, and attempts to memorize anything of worth proved fleeting at best. Thankfully, I have been blessed with superb teachers in my career (Drs. Ravi Lingam, J. Shenoy, and T.Y. Tan) who made this topic not only digestible but eventually immensely enjoyable too.

Temporal bone imaging like anything else in radiology becomes easier when one attains a sound anatomical footing, grasps the clinical scenario, and of course, PRACTICE!

This book has been designed with the trainee foremost in mind. The first section *"Basic anatomy and approach to common symptoms; making sense of history"* is intended to provide the reader an anatomical platform, overview of the available imaging modalities and concepts to the most commonly encountered clinical problems. The "approaches" for various symptoms explain relevant clinical findings, jargons, and will lay down a roadmap on how to arrive at the most likely diagnosis and plausible differentials. The subsequent sections will then provide a more detailed account of all the various pathologies seen in and around the temporal bone. All sections of the book include numerous "Tips," "Remember," and "What does the surgeon want to know" boxes that provide the reader with concise and relevant highlights for easy reference.

This book is my attempt at making a seemingly complex topic in radiology a tad easier for the trainee and the occasional reporter. It is by no means the complete work on temporal bone imaging but rather a survival handguide that should inspire further reading.

Singapore, Singapore
September 2020

Geoiphy George Pulickal

Acknowledgments

We would like to acknowledge the following people for their valuable contributions to this volume:

Professor Wilfred C. G. Peh (Khoo Teck Puat Hospital, Singapore) for his vision, constant encouragement, and editorial advice.

Dr. Ravi Lingam (Northwick Park & Central Middlesex Hospitals, London) for his imaging expertise, pictorial contributions, and caring mentorship.

Associate Professor Heng Wai Yuen (Changi General Hospital, Singapore), Dr. Alex Manoj Mathew (Khoo Teck Puat Hospital, Singapore), and Dr. Amanda Cheang (Woodlands Health Campus, Singapore) for dispensing their clinical expertise so readily and frequently.

About the Book

Temporal bone imaging is a complex and challenging topic in radiology. The delicate anatomy and unique pathology encountered in this region makes it a difficult terrain to master for radiologists and clinicians alike.

Written and edited by various experts in the field, this work is designed to be a handbook for the radiology and otorhinolaryngology trainee as well as the general radiologist, who has to report the occasional temporal bone study.

This work teaches practical temporal bone anatomy and guides the reader on how to approach common otological problems in a logical and systematic manner. All relevant pathology in and around the temporal bone are discussed in detail and illustrated with high quality examples in their respective sections. Emphasis is not only placed on diagnosis but also on how to differentiate important mimics and highlight vital surgical findings.

We have included numerous tips and memory boxes for easy reference throughout the book, to help the reader get a quick grasp of the topic and aid in forming a coherent and clinically relevant report.

Singapore   Geoiphy George Pulickal

Contents

Part I

Basic Anatomy and Approach to Common Symptoms; Making Sense of History

Basic Temporal Bone Imaging Anatomy: External, Middle and Inner Ear

Contents

Abstract

An understanding of the normal temporal bone anatomy is half the battle; in this chapter, a practical and relevant description of the anatomy is provided to enable the reader to better understand the subsequent pathology. The anatomy is broken down into various sub-sections, i.e. external, middle, inner ear and facial nerve. Simple illustrations and tables are provided that enable a more intuitive understanding of the complex anatomy and relationship between different anatomical structures. A glossary of various popular anatomical terms is provided for quick reference.

K. Chokkappan (✉)
Department of Diagnostic Radiology, Khoo Teck Puat Hospital, Singapore, Singapore
e-mail: chokkappan.kabilan@ktph.com.sg

© Springer Nature Switzerland AG 2021
G. G. Pulickal et al. (eds.), *Temporal Bone Imaging Made Easy*,
Medical Radiology Diagnostic Imaging, https://doi.org/10.1007/978-3-030-70635-7_1

1   Temporal Bone Overview

Temporal bones are a pair of skull bones that form the lateral skull base (Fig. 1 and Table 1). They contain several channels, intrinsic fissures and extrinsic sutures. Anatomically, the temporal bone consists of five distinct segments detailed below.

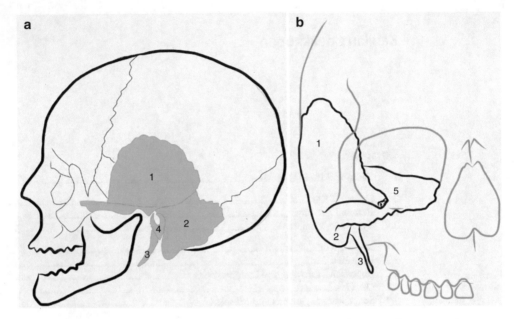

Fig. 1 (**a** and **b**) Gross anatomy of the temporal bone segments. (1) Squamous, (2) Mastoid, (3) Styloid, (4) Tympanic and (5) Petrous

Table 1 Segments of temporal bone

Segment	Description
Squamous	• Flat anterosuperior part • Articulates with parietal bone superiorly, greater wing of sphenoid anteriorly and rest of the temporal bone posteroinferiorly • Contains zygomatic process and mandibular fossa
Mastoid	• Posterior part with a cortical projection called mastoid process • Abuts parietal (superior) and occipital (posterior) bones
Styloid	• Long and slender projection from the inferior aspect of the temporal bone • Important landmark of neck compartments on cross-sectional imaging
Tympanic	• Curved plate of bone inferior to the squamous segment and anterior to the occipital bone • Forms the anterior, inferior and posterior walls of the external auditory canal (Fig. 2) • Gives attachment to the tympanic membrane
Petrous	• Wedge shaped bone mass projecting medially, lying between sphenoid and occipital bones in the skull base • Middle and inner ear is contained within the petrous temporal bone • Defines the axis of the temporal bone (especially in the context of trauma) • Consists of apex and base: – Apex: pointed medial aspect that forms the boundary of the carotid canal and foramen lacerum – Base: broad lateral aspect that merges with squamous segment • Contains three surfaces: – Anterior: Forms floor of the middle cranial fossa – Posterior: Forms anterior aspect of the posterior cranial fossa. Contains opening of the internal auditory canal and vestibular aqueduct – Inferior: Forms outer surface of the skull base. Contains structures such as carotid canal and jugular foramen

2 External Ear

The external ear consists of the pinna and the external auditory canal (EAC). The pinna is readily examined clinically and usually does not warrant any imaging.

2.1 External Ear Canal

The EAC is of more radiological concern, and it extends from the auricle to the tympanic membrane medially. The lateral one-third is fibrocartilaginous and medial is two-third osseous, formed by the tympanic portion of temporal bone (Fig. 2). The junction of the fibrocartilaginous and osseous segments forms a natural narrowing called the 'isthmus' (Fig. 3), and foreign bodies located medial to it are difficult to extract.

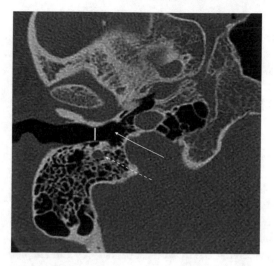

Fig. 3 Axial CT image just above the floor of the EAC. The isthmus of the EAC (white line) and the barely perceptible normal tympanic membrane (white arrow) are shown. The mastoid segment of the facial nerve (dashed arrow) surrounded by pneumatized mastoid air cells

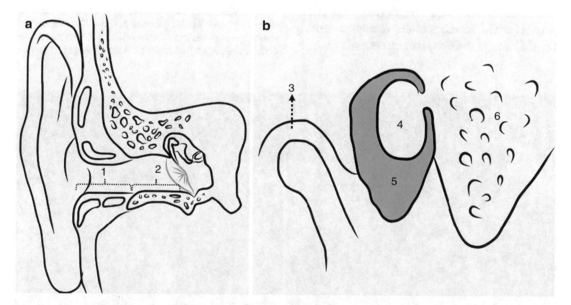

Fig. 2 (**a** and **b**) Coronal and sagittal illustrations of EAC. (1) Cartilaginous segment of the EAC, (2) Bony segment of the EAC, (3) Temporomandibular joint, (4) EAC, (5) Tympanic segment of the temporal bone and (6) Mastoid temporal bone

The anterior wall of the EAC forms the posterior aspect of the glenoid fossa (Fig. 3); hence, fractures of the EAC may extend to the temporomandibular joint. The posterior wall makes the anterior margin of the mastoid temporal bone and is removed during canal wall-down mastoidectomy (Fig. 3).

2.2　Tympanic Membrane

The tympanic membrane (TM) is located at the medial end of the EAC and separates the external ear from the middle ear. Under normal conditions, it is a translucent cone-like structure that points into the middle ear (refer Sect. 1 in chapter "Common Otoscopic Signs, Imaging of Common Surgeries and Implants") and is barely perceptible on CT (Fig. 3). The tip of the handle and lateral (short) process of the malleus are embedded upon it (Fig. 4). The anterior and posterior malleal folds divide the TM into the smaller pars flaccida superiorly and a larger pars tensa inferiorly. The TM attaches to the scutum superiorly (Fig. 5) and to the bony annulus elsewhere.

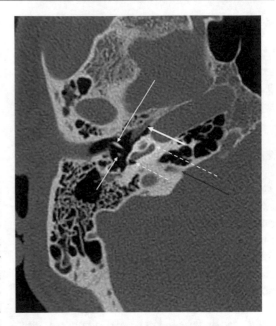

Fig. 4 Axial CT image showing the manubrium of the malleus (long white arrow) lying parallel to the long process of the incus (short white arrow). The round window (short-dashed arrow) lies immediately lateral to the basal turn of the cochlea (long dashed arrow). The belly of the tensor tympani muscle (short thick arrow) and part of the cochlear aqueduct (red arrow) are also seen at this level

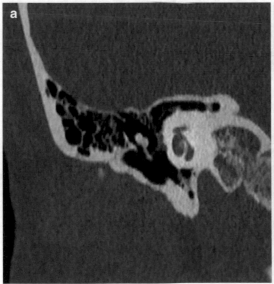

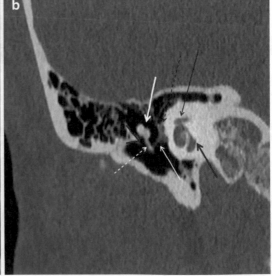

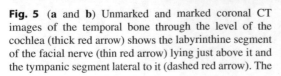

Fig. 5 (**a** and **b**) Unmarked and marked coronal CT images of the temporal bone through the level of the cochlea (thick red arrow) shows the labyrinthine segment of the facial nerve (thin red arrow) lying just above it and the tympanic segment lateral to it (dashed red arrow). The malleoincudal joint (thick white arrow) lies medial to the scutum (red outline) in the epitympanum, and the tensor tympani muscle (thin white arrow) inserts itself into the manubrium (dashed white arrow) of the malleus

3 Middle Ear

The middle ear or tympanic cavity is an air-filled space in the petrous temporal bone containing the ossicles and suspensory structures. It mainly functions as a means of impedance between the air-filled external ear and the fluid-filled inner ear in conducting the sound waves (Fig. 6). Its boundaries are described in Table 2.

3.1 Divisions

Middle ear is divided into three parts by its relationship with the tympanic membrane (Fig. 7 and Table 3), i.e. hypo, meso and epitympanum (below, at the level of and above the tympanic membrane).

Table 2 Boundaries of the middle ear

Boundaries/walls of the middle ear	Description/structures that form the boundaries
Lateral	Tympanic membrane
Medial	Inner ear structures contained in the otic capsule. Medial wall features the oval and round windows
Superior	Tegmen plate, thin plate of bone that separates the middle eat cavity from dura of the middle cranial fossa
Inferior	Jugular wall that separates the jugular bulb
Posterior	Contains the facial recess, pyramidal eminence (with stapedius muscle), sinus tympani and round window niche (in that order from lateral to medial). The aditus ad antrum lies in its superior part.
Anterior	Separates the middle ear from the carotid canal. Anterior wall has the opening of the Eustachian tube and the canal for the tensor tympani muscle

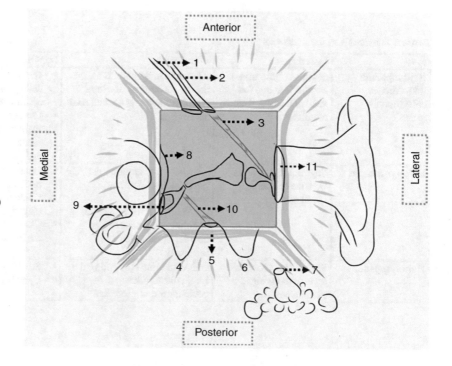

Fig. 6 The middle ear cavity as seen through the roof to demonstrate its relationship with the external and inner ear. Prominent structures in the anterior, posterior, medial and lateral walls are as follows, (1) Eustachian tube, (2) Canal for tensor tympani, (3) Tensor tympani tendon, (4) Sinus tympani, (5) Pyramidal eminence, (6) Facial recess, (7) Aditus ad antrum, (8) Cochlear promontory, (9) Oval window, (10) Stapedius and (11) Tympanic membrane

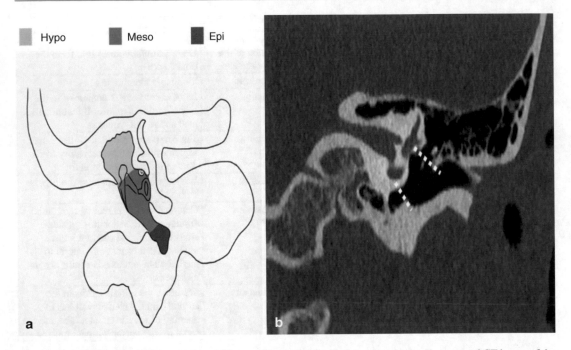

Fig. 7 (**a** and **b**) Divisions of the middle ear illustrated coronal right ear (**a**) and corresponding coronal CT image of the left ear (**b**) with dotted lines representing the superior and inferior margins of the TM

Table 3 Divisions of the middle ear

Parts	Description	Boundaries	Important notes
Epitympanum (aka Attic or epitympanic recess)	Segment of the middle ear that is above the level of the tympanic membrane	Above an imaginary line drawn between scutum and tympanic segment of the facial nerve (Fig. 8)	• Connects to the mastoid air cells posteriorly via the *aditus ad antrum* (Figs. 9 and 10) • Contains the head of the malleus, the body and short process of the incus (Figs. 8, 9 and 23)
Mesotympanum	Segment that is level with the tympanic membrane	Line between scutum to tympanic facial nerve superiorly Line between the tympanic annulus to the base of the cochlear promontory inferiorly	• Contains the rest of the ossicular chain • Contains the tensor tympani (Fig. 4) and stapedius muscles • Chorda tympani nerve traverses the mesotympanum
Hypotympanum	Part that is below the level of the tympanic membrane	Below the line connecting the tympanic annulus and cochlear promontory base	• Smallest division • Opening of the Eustachian tube

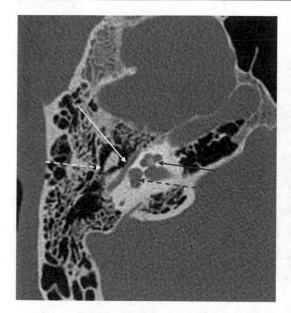

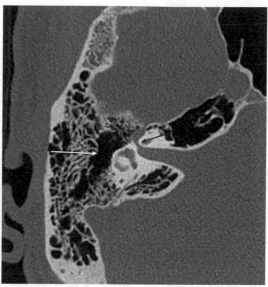

Fig. 8 Axial CT image showing the tympanic segment of the facial nerve (white arrow), the short process of the incus (white dashed arrow) pointing into the incudal fossa, the modiolus (red arrow) and part of the vestibule (red dashed arrow)

Fig. 10 Axial CT image through the epitympanum depicting the labyrinthine segment of the facial nerve (red arrow), geniculate ganglion (red dashed arrow) and the superior part of the aditus ad antrum (white arrow)

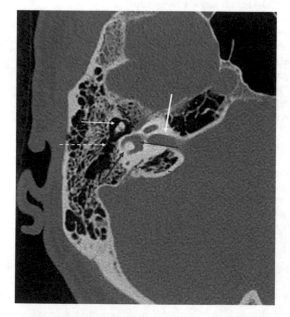

Fig. 9 Axial CT image through the epitympanum depicting the normal malleo-incudal articulation in partial 'ice cream cone' configuration (white arrow) and the aditus ad antrum (dashed white arrow). The lateral semi-circular canal (thick red arrow) communicates with the vestibule (red arrow). Part of IAC (thick white arrow) and vestibular aqueduct (red dashed arrow) are appreciated at this level as well

3.2   Important Structures and Landmarks (Table 4)

Table 4 Middle ear - important landmarks

Structures	Description
Scutum	• Sharp bony projection from the medial aspect of roof of the EAC, where the tympanic membrane attaches superiorly. It forms the lateral boundary of the Prussak space and is best demonstrated in the coronal images (Fig. 5). Erosion or blunting of the scutum is one of the earliest signs of pars flaccida (acquired) cholesteatoma
Prussak space	• Prussak space (Fig. 11) is a small space within the larger lateral epitympanic space bounded by the pars flaccida of the tympanic membrane laterally, neck of the malleus medially, lateral malleal ligament superiorly and lateral process of the malleus inferiorly • Pars flaccida cholesteatoma generally begins here and erodes into the adjacent structures like the ossicles and scutum
Oval window (fenestra vestibuli)	• Small oval communication between the mesotympanic middle ear and the vestibule of the inner ear (Figs. 12 and 13) • Stapes footplate closes the window with its rim covered by the annular ligament
Round window	• Another natural opening/window between the middle and the inner ear (Fig. 4) • Covered by a thin pseudo-membrane, infrequently visible on imaging • During sound transmission, the inward motion of the oval window/stapes footplate is accompanied by outward motion of the secondary tympanic membrane, resulting in movement of the perilymph • Stenosis or atresia results in conductive hearing loss
Round window niche	• Is a recess partially covered by a thin overhanging bone arising from the promontory that may obscure the niche and round window during surgery (Fig. 14), hence the importance of radiological assessment preoperatively
Fissula ante-fenestram (cochlear cleft)	• Small cleft filled with connective tissue located immediately anterior to the oval window and posterior to the cochleariform process (Fig. 12) • Most common site of origin of fenestral otosclerosis
Pyramidal eminence	• Hollow bony projection from the posterior wall of the middle ear (Fig. 15) • Lies between the sinus tympani medially and the facial recess laterally (Fig. 15) • The stapedius muscle originates from the central hole at the apex of the eminence
Auditory (Eustachian) tube	• Connects the tympanic cavity with the nasopharynx (Fig. 16) • Consists of bony one-third extending from the anterior wall of the middle ear and cartilaginous two-third opening into the nasopharynx • Helps in equalizing intra-tympanic pressure with the atmospheric pressure and mucociliary clearance of the tympanic cavity
Mastoid air cells	• Cluster of air cells contained in the mastoid temporal bone (Fig. 3) • Located posterior to the epitympanum • Mastoid antrum (Fig. 17) is the largest air cell that communicates with epitympanic middle ear via aditus • Buffers middle ear during eustachian tube dysfunction to combat negative pressure • Potential source/reservoir of recurrent middle ear infection

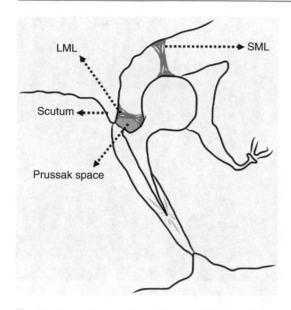

Fig. 11 Prussak space (shaded in grey). *LML* lateral malleal ligament, *SML* superior malleal ligament

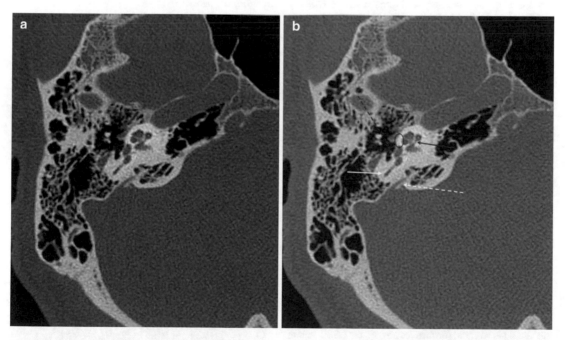

Fig. 12 (**a** and **b**) Unmarked and marked axial CT images of temporal bone showing part of the posterior semi-circular canal (white arrow) and a normal calibre vestibular aqueduct (dashed white arrow) containing the endolymphatic duct. The stapes (red dashed arrow) articulating with the oval window and the fissula ante fenstram (red oval outline) lies anterior to it. The modiolus of the cochlea (red arrow) is partially seen

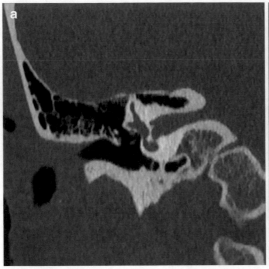 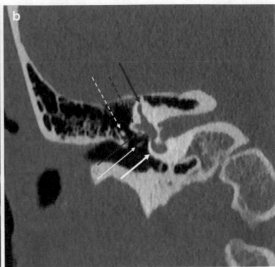

Fig. 13 (**a** and **b**) Unmarked and marked coronal CT images through the level of the IAM shows the tympanic segment of the facial nerve (thin red arrow) lying just below the lateral semi-circular canal (LSCC) (red dashed arrow), and the superior semi-circular canal (SSCC) (thick red arrow) lies perpendicular to the LSCC. The oval window (red line) lies above the cochlear promontory (thick white arrow). The head of the stapes (thin white arrow) can be seen facing the oval window, and the tip of the short process of the malleus (dashed white arrow) lies in the epitympanum

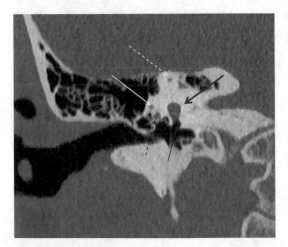 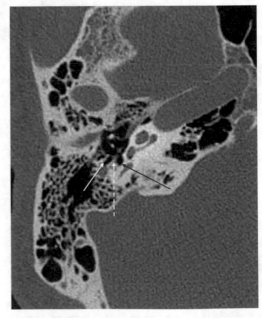

Fig. 14 Coronal CT image through the level of the vestibule (thick red arrow) shows the partly covered round window niche (thin red arrow), the tympanic segment of the facial nerve canal (dashed red arrow), the LSSC (white arrow) and SSCC (dashed white arrow)

Fig. 15 Axial CT image showing the pyramidal eminence (dashed white arrow) from which the stapedius muscle originates. The sinus tympani (red arrow) lies medial and the facial nerve recess lateral to the pyramidal eminence (white arrow)

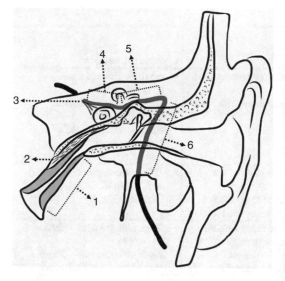

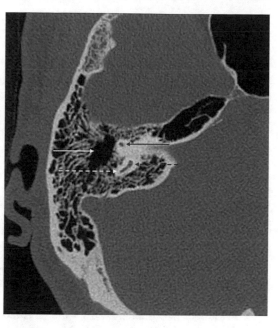

Fig. 16 Illustration demonstrating auditory tube and facial nerve in the middle ear. (1) Cartilaginous portion of the Eustachian tube, (2) Tensor tympani muscle, (3) Internal acoustic meatus, (4) Labyrinthine VII N, (5) Tympanic VII N and (6) Mastoid VII N

Fig. 17 Axial CT image depicting the anterior limb of the superior semi-circular canal (red arrow), part of the medial limb of the posterior semi-circular canal (dashed white arrow) that forms part of the common crus (red dashed arrow). The mastoid antrum (white arrow) is the largest mastoid air cell

Fig. 18 Ossicular chain and suspensory apparatus. *TT* tensor tympani, *AML* anterior malleal ligament, *SML* Superior malleal ligament, *SIL* superior incudal ligament, *PIL* posterior incudal ligament

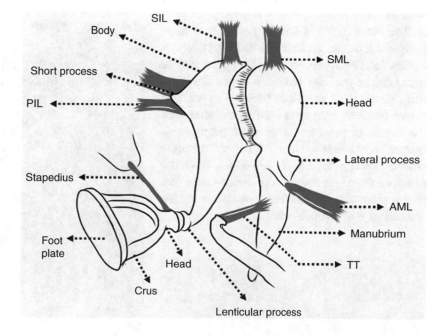

3.3 Ossicles

The ossicles form a chain of three small inter-articulating bones extending from the tympanic membrane to the oval window, conducting sound vibrations to the inner ear (Fig. 18 and Table 5). Knowledge on various parts of the ossicles and appearance of their normal articulations helps in identifying subtle ossicular dysplasia, erosions and trauma-related injuries.

Table 5 Ossicular chain and suspensory apparatus

Ossicles (lateral to medial)	Parts of ossicles	Articulation	Ligaments/muscles
Malleus	Head, neck, anterior process, lateral process and manubrium	• Manubrium of the malleus attaches to the tympanic membrane • Head of the malleus articulates with body of the incus	• AML → Head to anterior tympanic wall • LML → Neck to lateral tympanic wall • SML → Head to roof of tympanic cavity • Tensor tympani → manubrium
Incus	Body, short process, long process and lenticular process	• Head of the malleus with body of the incus (malleoincudal joint) • Lenticular process of the incus with the head of the stapes (incudostapedial joint)	• PIL → Short process of incus to the incudal fossa (fossa incudes) (Fig. 8)
Stapes	head/capitellum, anterior crus, posterior crus and footplate	• Lenticular process of the incus with the head of the stapes (incudostapedial joint) • Stapes footplates attach to the oval window via the annular ligament (Fig. 12)	• Stapedius muscle → head of the stapes • Annular ligament → Stapes foot plate to the oval window

The malleus (hammer in Latin) is the most lateral ossicle and articulates with the tympanic membrane via its manubrium (aka as handle) and the lateral process. The anterior malleal ligament attaches itself to the malleus via a small projection at its neck called the anterior process. The posterior margin of the malleus head articulates with the incus.

The incus (anvil in Latin) consists of a large body that articulates with the malleus and two processes, i.e. a short process and a long process. The distal end of the long process is called the lentiform process that articulates with the stapes. The stapes (meaning stirrup in Latin) articulates with the lentiform process via its head (capitulum). Immediately below the head the stapedius muscle attaches itself to the neck of the stapes. From the neck two crura – anterior and posterior – arise that attach themselves to the footplate which in turn articulates with the oval window.

> **Tip**
> *On axial section, the following imaging signs can be used to identify the normal alignment of the ossicles:*
>
> - *'Two parallel lines' formed by handle of malleus anteriorly and long process of incus posteriorly (Fig. 4)*

> - *'Two dots' formed by the head of stapes medially and the lenticular process of incus laterally (Fig. 19)*
> - *'Ice cream cone' appearance formed by the malleoincudal joint (Fig. 9)*

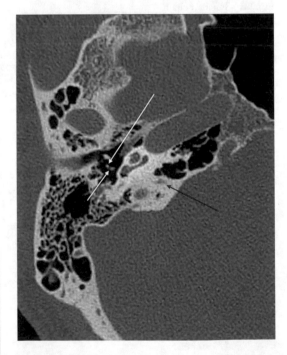

Fig. 19 Axial CT image showing the lenticular process of incus (long white arrow) and the head of the stapes (short white arrow) as two aligned dots. The cochlear aqueduct is partially seen (red arrow)

3.4 Suspensory Ligaments and Muscles

Tendons of the tensor tympani and stapedius muscles and various suspensory ligaments help stabilize the ossicular chain. Unfortunately, these structures have varying ranges of visibility on CT and are often difficult to discern. The anterior, lateral, and superior malleal ligaments and the posterior incudal ligament attach the malleus and incus to the walls of the middle ear (Fig. 18 and Table 5). Undue prominence of the suspensory ligaments, calcification, or absence of normally seen ligaments could be the cause of conductive hearing loss and should be looked for in appropriate clinical context (e.g. tympanosclerosis).

Tensor tympani and stapedius muscles have protective function as they help dampen the loud low-pitch noise and vibrations from reaching the inner ear. Tensor tympani originates from the cartilaginous portion of the eustachian tube and inserts into the neck of the malleus. It is supplied by the nerve for tensor tympani, a branch of mandibular nerve. Stapedius muscle is the smallest muscle in the body. It arises from the apex of the pyramidal eminence and inserts into the neck of the stapes. It is innervated by facial nerve.

4 Inner Ear

Inner ear consists of bony and membranous labyrinth (Fig. 20) and is contained within the petrous temporal bone. It is responsible for hearing, balance and equilibrium. Naturally, the bony labyrinth is better assessed with CT, whereas the fluid-filled spaces of the inner ear are better seen with MRI.

Bony labyrinth is comprised of the cochlea, vestibule and three semi-circular canals (lateral, posterior and superior) (Figs. 4, 5, 8, 9, 10, 12, 13, 14, 15 and 19). The thickened part of the temporal bone around the bony labyrinth is known as otic capsule. The bony labyrinth contains the perilymph in which the membranous labyrinth is suspended.

Membranous labyrinth (Fig. 20) is an actual structure that cannot be separately visualized on CT and contains endolymph. Its anatomy conforms to that of the bony labyrinth except for the two small sacs, the utricle and saccule, that are contained within the bony vestibule. The utricle communicates posteriorly with the semi-circular ducts via five orifices and anteriorly with the saccule by the utriculosaccular duct. The saccule gives opening for the endolymphatic duct in its posterior wall.

Fig. 20 Illustration of inner ear, membranous labyrinth shaded in grey

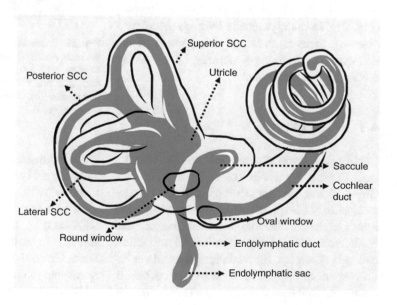

Fig. 21 Illustration of the cochlea

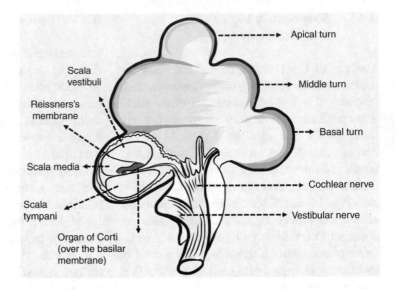

The Scala media (aka cochlear duct or ductus cochlearis) is an endolymph-containing structure that lies between the perilymph containing Scala vestibuli (above) and Scala tympani (below). Its floor is formed by the basilar membrane, and the roof is formed by the vestibular or Reissner's membrane. Scala media hosts the organ of Corti, which is the terminal 'unit of hearing' containing thousands of auditory nerve receptors and their hair cells that help to transform the mechanical vibration of sound into electrical signals in the process of hearing (Fig. 21). In endolymphatic hydrops (Meniere's disease), there is abnormal enlargement of the endolymph-containing structures, i.e. the Scala media, utricle and saccule.

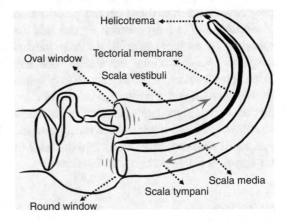

Fig. 22 Schematic representation of fluid dynamics in the inner ear. Inward displacement of foot plate in the oval window is accompanied displacement of the round window membrane in the opposite direction, resulting in movement of perilymph and subsequently the endolymph

4.1   Cochlea

Cochlea is a spiral structure that makes about 2.5 (to 2.7) turns around its axis called the modiolus (Figs. 12 and 15). An incomplete thin bony septum, namely the spiral lamina, separates the spiral lumen of the cochlea into two, Scala tympani and Scala vestibuli. At the apex of the modiolus, called helicotrema, the Scala tympani and vestibuli meet each other. The basal turn of cochlea is connected to the middle ear at the round window.

There is inward displacement of the oval window and outward bulge of the membrane covering the round window, as the sound waves reach the foot plate of stapes and travel along the fluid in the inner ear (Fig. 22). The cochlear aqueduct (Figs. 4 and 19) is a small linear channel that connects the Scala tympani to the subarachnoid space, as it opens into the inferior wall of the petrous temporal bone lateral to the jugular foramen.

4.2 Vestibule

Vestibule (Figs. 8, 9 and 14) is the oval central part of the labyrinth that contains utricle and saccule of the membranous labyrinth. It contains the oval window in its lateral wall and spherical and elliptical recesses corresponding to saccule and utricle in the medial wall. Openings of the semi-circular canals and vestibular aqueduct (Fig. 8) are also seen in the vestibule. The vestibular aqueduct contains the endolymphatic duct that ends in a blind pouch called endolymphatic sac posteriorly between the layers of the dura. The duct and the sac contain the endolymph and play a role in the metabolic activity of the inner ear. Enlarged vestibular aqueduct (measuring more than 1.5 mm diameter in the mid-segment) is a sign of endolymphatic sac dysfunction and can be seen in inner ear abnormalities associated with hearing loss.

> **Tip**
> • *As a rule, the endolymphatic duct should never be thicker than any of the posterior semi-circular canal*

4.3 Semi-circular Canals

Three semi-circular canals, namely the superior (Fig. 17), lateral (Fig. 9) and posterior (Fig. 12), form the posterior part of the inner ear. The bony canals measure about 1 mm in diameter and are arranged approximately perpendicular to each other. The superior covering of the superior semi-circular canal forms the arcuate eminence in the roof of the petrous temporal bone (important in cases of dehiscence). The part of the lateral semi-circular canal, where it normally projects into the epitympanic cavity laterally, is prone to erosion from cholesteatomas resulting in endolymphatic fistula. Each canal has a non-dilated end on one side and a dilated end on the other called an ampulla. The non-ampullary end of the superior and posterior canals forms a common crus (Fig. 17) and opens into the vestibule.

4.4 Internal Acoustic Meatus

The internal acoustic meatus (or internal auditory canal—IAC) is a bony canal in the posterior wall of the petrous temporal bone that carries the seventh and eighth nerves as they enter and exit the brainstem. Porus acousticus is the lateral wider end of the IAC, whereas the medial end that abuts the labyrinth is called the fundus. A thin transverse bony structure called crista falciformis divides the IAC into superior and inferior compartments. A partial vertical Bills bar separates the superior compartment into anterior and posterior compartments. The facial and cochlear nerves are located in the anterosuperior and anteroinferior compartments, respectively [mnemonic clue 'Seven (cranial nerve VII) Up/Coke (cochlear nerve) down]. The superior and inferior vestibular nerves are in the superoposterior and inferoposterior compartments, respectively (Fig. 23).

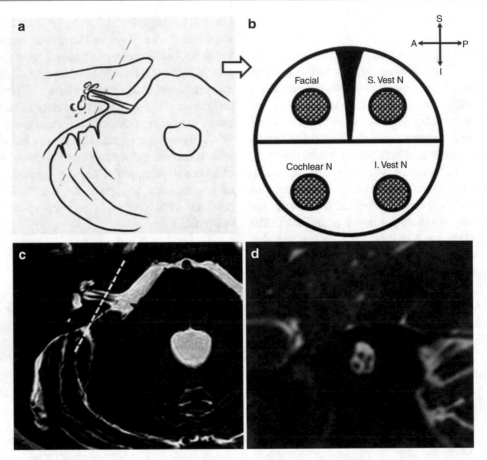

Fig. 23 (**a** and **b**) Diagrams showing arrangement of the VII and VIII nerve complex in the internal auditory canal. The facial nerve occupies the anterosuperior quadrant, the cochlear nerve the anteroinferior quadrant, and the ves- tibular nerves the posterior aspect of the IAC. (**c** and **d**) Corresponding axial and oblique sagittal highly T2-weighted fluid-sensitive 3D MR images showing the anatomic relationship

5   Facial Nerve

Knowing the course of the facial nerve and anat- omy of its bony canal helps in the assessment of the facial nerve (Fig. 24). The facial nerve is divided into various segments as enumerated below (Table 6). Often, oblique reconstruction helps provide a more complete view of the facial nerve (refer Sect. 1 in chapter "Temporal Bone imaging techniques: Computer Tomography, Cone Beam CT and Magnetic Resonance Imaging").

> **Tip**
> - *Faint enhancement of geniculate gan- glion, tympanic and mastoid segments of facial nerve on MR is considered nor- mal; everything else is abnormal.*

Fig. 24 Illustration of the various cranial nerve segments in the temporal bone

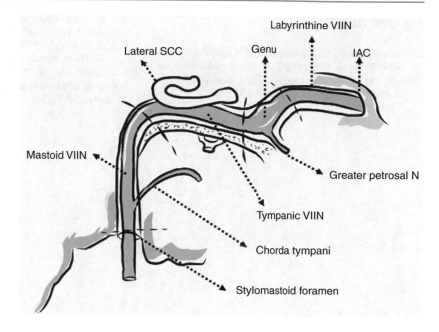

Table 6 Segments of the facial nerve

Segment	Description	Imaging anatomy	Branches
Cisternal	Arising from the anterolateral aspect of the pons to the porus acousticus of IAC	• Runs anterior to CN VIII • Best assessed on fluid-sensitive high-resolution T2 images (Fig. 23)	No Branches
Intra-canalicular	Segment within the IAC, from Porus acousticus to fundus of IAC	• Anterior superior quadrant of the IAC • Best assessed on the oblique sagittal high-resolution T2 images (Fig. 23)	No Branches
Labyrinthine	From entry into the fallopian canal (facial nerve canal) till the geniculate ganglion	• Shortest and narrowest segment • Anterior to the cochlea (Fig. 10) • Coronal section: Look for the 'snake eyes' (Fig. 5) made by the labyrinthine and proximal tympanic segments	Greater superficial petrosal nerve (GSPN), lesser petrosal and external petrosal nerves
Tympanic	From geniculate ganglion to posterior genu of facial nerve	• Horizontal course along the medial wall of the middle ear (Fig. 8) • Coronal sections: inferior to the lateral SCC and superolateral to oval window (Fig. 13)	No Branches
Mastoid	From posterior genu to stylomastoid mastoid foramen	• Vertical course just behind the EAC till it exits the skull (Fig. 3)	Nerve to stapedius and Chorda tympani
Extra-cranial	Beyond the stylomastoid foramen into the parotid space	• The plane of the traversing facial nerve divides the parotid gland into superficial and deep parts	Five terminal branches—temporal, zygomatic, buccal, mandibular and cervical

Further Reading

Juliano AF, Ginat DT, Moonis G (2013) Imaging review of the temporal bone: part I. Anatomy and inflammatory and neoplastic processes. Radiology 269(1):17–33. https://doi.org/10.1148/radiol.13120733

Juliano AF (2018) Cross sectional imaging of the ear and temporal bone. Head Neck Pathol 12(3):302–320. https://doi.org/10.1007/s12105-018-0901-y

Lemmerling MM, Stambuk HE, Mancuso AA, Antonelli PJ, Kubilis PS (1997) CT of the normal suspensory ligaments of the ossicles in the middle ear. AJNR Am J Neuroradiol 18(3):471–477

Temporal Bone Imaging Techniques: Computer Tomography, Cone Beam CT and Magnetic Resonance Imaging

Geoiphy George Pulickal

Contents

Abstract

This chapter provides an overview of the available temporal bone imaging modalities, their specific uses and limitations. Basic scanning protocol principles for each modality are explained. Common multiplanar reconstructions are demonstrated, and stepwise instructions are provided on how to obtain them.

1 Radiographs

Historically, plain radiographs did play a limited role in assessing the degree of mastoid pneumatisation, detection of lytic bone lesions etc. In the current era of digital imaging, radiographs do not serve any meaningful role apart from assessing the position and integrity of cochlea implants (refer Sect. 1 in chapter 'Common Otoscopic Signs, Imaging of Common Surgeries and Implants').

2 Multi-detector Computer Tomography

Multi-detector computer tomography (CT) of the temporal bone is easily available and cost-effective. It allows for volumetric acquisition from which the desired high-resolution coronal and axial reconstructions are obtained.

Axial planes are obtained in a plane parallel to the lateral semi-circular canal (LSCC). This is achieved by going through the sagittal data set and finding the image, where both the anterior and the posterior limbs of the LSSC are seen; the plane connecting these two limbs (Fig. 1) will yield an axial plane, where the lateral SSC is visible in its

G. G. Pulickal (✉)
Department of Diagnostic Radiology, Khoo Teck Puat Hospital, Singapore, Singapore
e-mail: pulickal.george.geoiphy@ktph.com.sg

© Springer Nature Switzerland AG 2021
G. G. Pulickal et al. (eds.), *Temporal Bone Imaging Made Easy*,
Medical Radiology Diagnostic Imaging, https://doi.org/10.1007/978-3-030-70635-7_2

entirety (Fig. 1). Coronal planes are then reconstructed perpendicular to this acquired axial plane.

These planes should be obtained in bone windows/algorithms with sub-millimetre thickness (0.3 or 0.6 mm) being essential. Axial coverage must include the top of the petrous apex cranially and the tip of the mastoid caudally. Coronal coverage must at least commence anterior to the facial geniculate ganglion and extend to the posterior margin of the mastoid.

Additional soft tissue windows can be reconstructed in thicker slices (2 mm). Use of intravenous contrast (e.g. for suspected malignancy or deep-seated infection etc.) should be limited only to specific instances or when MR imaging is not possible.

Numerous popular reformats are available to highlight different parts of the temporal bone anatomy, e.g. the Poschl projection for the superior semi-circular canal (SSCC) (refer Sect. 4 in chapter 'Other Causes of Inner Ear Hearing Loss: Meniere's Disease, Labyrinthitis and Semicircular Canal Dehiscence') or oblique reformations to visualise the tympanic and mastoid segments of the facial nerve on a single image (Fig. 2). The

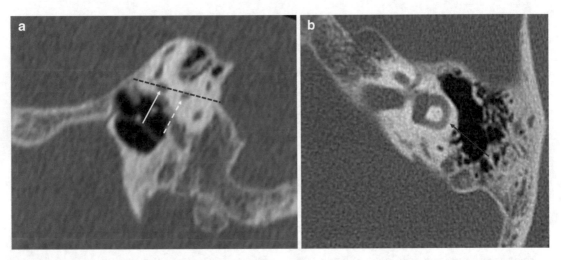

Fig. 1 (**a** and **b**) Reference sagittal scout image showing the anterior (white arrow) and posterior (white dashed arrow) limbs of the lateral semi-circular canal, the axial plane is reformatted in the plane dissecting through them (dashed red line). Resultant axial image will show the lateral semi-circular canal in its entirety (red arrow)

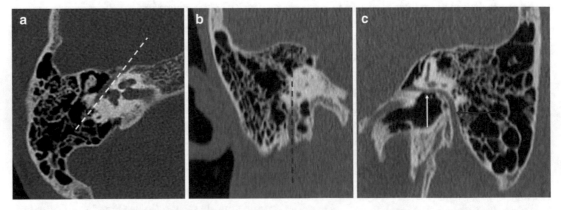

Fig. 2 (**a–c**) Double oblique reconstructions along the tympanic segment of facial nerve on the axial plane (dashed white line) and along the mastoid segment on the coronal plane (dashed red line) are needed to visualize the facial nerve better. Oblique reconstruction along these planes allows for more complete assessment of the tympanic (white arrow) and mastoid (red arrow) segments of the facial nerve

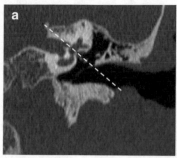 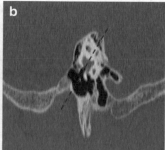 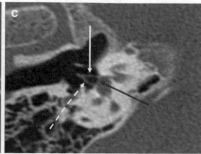

Fig. 3 (**a–c**) Double oblique reconstruction along the stapes through the oval window on the coronal (dashed white line) and sagittal (dashed red line) planes allows for better visualization of both the anterior (white arrow) and posterior (dashed white arrow) stapes crura as well as the stapes footplate (red arrow)

Stenver plane is perpendicular to the Poschl plane and is used in trauma assessment. Some relationships such as the stapes-oval window are better seen on double oblique reconstructions (Fig. 3).

3   Cone Beam X-Ray Computer Tomography (CBCT)

CBCT is a relatively new CT technology that provided excellent spatial resolution for high-density structures at low radiation doses (Table 1). An entire 3D set of the images can be acquired by a single rotation of a gantry (to which an X-ray tube and detector are attached). The 'cone-shaped' X-ray beam is focused upon the temporal bone, and all necessary reconstructions can be derived from the 3D set.

> **Tip**
> • *CBCT provides better assessment of surgical implants over conventional MDCT, given the reduced metallic artefacts.*

4   Magnetic Resonance Imaging (MRI)

MRI imaging of the temporal bones should be reserved for assessment of the inner ear structures and diagnosis of cholesteatoma (if conventional CT imaging proves inconclusive). MRI in

Table 1 Cone Beam CT overview

Pro	Con
High spatial resolution	High susceptibility to motion artefacts
Low radiation doses	Poor assessment of soft tissue structures
Reduced metallic artefacts	Lack of widespread availability
Increased patient comfort (upright positioning and quick examination time)	

malignant otitis externa is usually done to assess intracranial complication rather than the temporal bones per se (refer Sect. 2 in chapter 'Radiological Features of Otitis Externa').

Assessment of the inner ear could either be a simple screening study comprising usually of a heavily T2-weighted 3D sequence (e.g. CISS sequence on a Siemens scanner or FIESTA sequence on GE) (Fig. 4) through the cerebello-pontine angles or a more complex multi-planar pre- and post-contrast study when a space-occupying lesion is suspected.

Non-echo planar imaging (Non-EPI) DWI with its reduced artefacts and better spatial resolution is gaining increased popularity in post-operative cholesteatoma imaging by detecting recurrent or residual disease, often negating the need for second-look surgery (refer Sect. 3 in chapter 'Radiological Features of Acquired and Congenital Cholesteatoma').

Another specific role for MRI is in the imaging of endolymphatic hydrops, where MRI is able to demonstrate the abnormal enlargement of

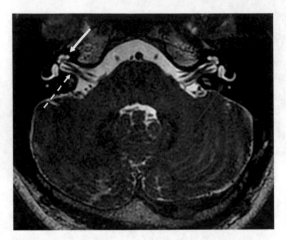

Fig. 4 Heavily T2-weighted 3D sequence through the cerebello-pontine angles provides exquisite visualization of the 7/8th nerve complex (white dashed arrow), cochlea (white arrow) and semi-circular canals (red arrow)

the endolymph-containing structures of the membranous labyrinth (refer Sect. 4 in chapter 'Other Causes of Inner Ear Hearing Loss: Meniere's Disease, Labyrinthitis and Semi-circular Canal Dehiscence').

Further Reading

Abele TA, Wiggins RH 3rd (2015) Imaging of the temporal bone. Radiol Clin N Am 53(1):15–36. https://doi.org/10.1016/j.rcl.2014.09.010. Review

Lane JI, Lindell EP, Witte RJ, DeLone DR, Driscoll CL (2006) Middle and inner ear: improved depiction with multiplanar reconstruction of volumetric CT data. Radiographics 26(1):115–124. Review

Miracle AC, Mukherji SK (2009) Conebeam CT of the head and neck, part 1: physical principles. AJNR Am J Neuroradiol 30(6):1088–1095. https://doi.org/10.3174/ajnr.A1653. Epub 2009 May 13. Review

Miracle AC, Mukherji SK (2009) Conebeam CT of the head and neck, part 2: clinical applications. AJNR Am J Neuroradiol 30(7):1285–1292. https://doi.org/10.3174/ajnr.A1654. Epub 2009 May 20. Review

Más-Estellés F, Mateos-Fernández M, Carrascosa-Bisquert B, Facal de Castro F, Puchades-Román I, Morera-Pérez C (2012) Contemporary non-echoplanar diffusion-weighted imaging of middle ear cholesteatomas. Radiographics 32(4):1197–1213. https://doi.org/10.1148/rg.324115109

Imaging Approach to Conductive Hearing Loss

Geoiphy George Pulickal

Contents

Abstract

The reasons for conductive hearing loss are extremely varied. This chapter explains how to utilise relevant clinical history and findings to narrow down potential causes. Details on how to review the cross-sectional imaging in a systematic manner to avoid any misses and highlight the relevant pathology are provided.

1 What Is Conductive Hearing Loss (CHL)

CHL is the disruption of sound conduction from the external world to the cochlea. This disruption can happen anywhere along the path of sound conduction.

2 Relevant Clinical Information

Audiometry and otoscopic findings will help narrow down the differentials.

2.1 Audiometry

The affected ear will show an elevated hearing threshold for air conduction and normal

G. G. Pulickal (✉)
Department of Diagnostic Radiology, Khoo Teck Puat Hospital, Singapore, Singapore
e-mail: pulickal.george.geoiphy@ktph.com.sg

© Springer Nature Switzerland AG 2021
G. G. Pulickal et al. (eds.), *Temporal Bone Imaging Made Easy*,
Medical Radiology Diagnostic Imaging, https://doi.org/10.1007/978-3-030-70635-7_3

threshold for bone conduction, and this difference is referred to as an increased air-bone gap.

2.2 Otoscopic Findings

Classical otoscopic findings mentioned in the imaging request history often provide the diagnosis itself or at least narrows the differentials considerably, e.g. acute otitis media or glomus tympanicum (refer Sect. 1 in chapter "Common Otoscopic Signs, Imaging of Common Surgeries and Implants").

3 Choice of Imaging

An unenhanced high-resolution CT scan of the temporal bone should be the first line of imaging. MRI only has a supportive role in CHL.

4 Assessment Pathway

We recommend a systematic approach analysing for structural abnormality, laterally to medially, i.e. external ear to oval and round windows, following the conduction of sound (Fig. 1).

4.1 External Ear Canal (EAC)

Typical clinical findings often help in reaching the diagnosis, e.g. the presence of squames and erosions point to an EAC cholesteatoma, granulation tissue in a diabetic patient raises suspicion for malignant otitis externa (MOE), presence of a pseudo-fundus may indicate underlying medial canal fibrosis (MCF) etc. Congenital atresia of the EAC is diagnosed clinically, and imaging is

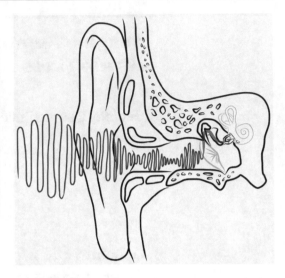

Fig. 1 Pathway of sound conduction. (Illustrated by Dr. Kabilan Chokkappan, Singapore)

performed to assess the associated abnormalities (refer Sect. 2 in chapter "Imaging of External Ear Malformations, Canal Stenosis and Exostosis").

Assess the calibre of the EAC and its bony margins; is it smoothly expanded (diffuse or focal), eroded, narrowed or occluded?

4.2 Middle Ear

The first task is to assess whether the middle ear cleft (MEC) is well pneumatised or not.

If the MEC is sclerosed (under pneumatised) and opacified, then the cause is usually acute or chronic otomastoiditis (refer Sect. 3 chapter "Imaging of Otomastoiditis, Acute and Chronic"), and a history of otorrhea will invariably be present.

The well-pneumatised MEC provides a difficult diagnostic challenge and requires a stepwise assessment from tympanic membrane to the oval and round windows.

4.2.1 Tympanic Membrane

The normal TM should barely be perceptible on CT imaging. Any subtle thickening or sclerosis may impede sound transmission and could indicate myringosclerosis (usually post-inflammatory or due to prior instrumentation, tympanoplasty).

4.2.2 Ossicular Chain (OC)

Any defect or misalignment of the OC, i.e. malleus, incus or stapes results in CHL.

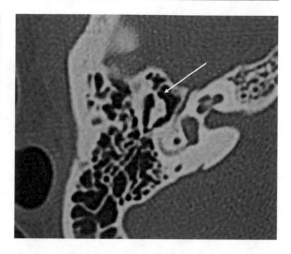

Fig. 2 Axial CT image shows fixation of the malleus to the lateral tympanic wall via an ossified anterior malleal ligament (arrow)

4.2.2.1 Malformations
Usually congenital and diagnosed in childhood. Hypoplasia of any ossicular bone (partial or complete) commonly involves the stapes or long process of incus. Look for ossicular fusion and fixation, e.g. malleus to the tympanic wall (Fig. 2).

4.2.2.2 Discontinuity
Dislocations are usually traumatic in nature and associated with fractures; five types have been recognized (refer Sect. 5 in chapter "Imaging of Temporal Bone Trauma"). The incus has the least ligamentous support hence the most involved.

Assess for discontinuity in the chain, the long process of incus is most commonly affected, usually post-inflammatory, traumatic, congenital or related to aging. If the OC has been reconstructed, then evaluate for prosthetic dislocations/subluxation.

4.2.2.3 Fixations

Post-inflammatory soft tissue along the ossicles impedes their movement, often a difficult diagnosis as this soft tissue can resemble fluid or granulation tissue. **Tympanosclerosis**, i.e. abnormal calcification along OC, muscles and ligaments is slightly more specific (refer Sect. 3 in chapter "Imaging of Otomastoiditis, Acute and Chronic").

Rare causes of ossicular fixation (impeding movement) include a persistent stapedial artery or a protruding facial nerve impeding the stapes (Fig. 3).

4.2.3 Oval and Round Windows

The oval window (OW) is an opening along the mesotympanum that transmits sound vibrations from the middle ear to the inner ear cochlea. The stapes footplate attaches to the OW via the annular ligament. The round window is another middle ear opening that dispels the build pressure in the cochlea from the transmitted sound vibrations.

As such, anything that prevents sound transmissions through the OW or dissipation through the round window can cause CHL.

– Stapes footplate fixation: new bone formation in Otosclerosis (refer Sect. 4 in chapter "Radiological Features of Otosclerosis")
– Oval window atresia: childhood presentation with CHL or mixed hearing loss (refer Sect. 3 in chapter "Radiological Features of Oval Window Atresia")
– Round window occlusion: usually due to middle ear lesions such as cholesteatoma, otitis media or otosclerosis but can also be due to anatomical variants such as a high-riding jugular bulb (Fig. 4).

4.2.4 Rare Causes

Some causes unfortunately do not fit into the above-mentioned systematic review. Causes such as temporal bone dysplasia, e.g. fibrous dysplasia, Paget's disease (Fig. 5), osteoporosis etc. are readily visible and usually not a diagnostic dilemma.

A mixed type of hearing loss could indicate third-window phenomenon that refers to sound dissipation through openings other than the oval or round windows e.g. superior semicircular canal dehiscence, enlarged vestibular aqueduct, cochlea dehiscence etc. This requires a closer look at these sites (refer Sect. 4 in chapter "Other Causes of

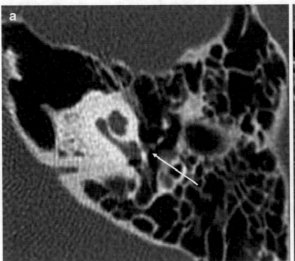
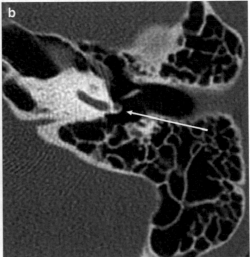

Fig. 3 (**a** and **b**) Axial CT image through the level of the stapes (**a**) shows a persistent stapedial artery as a focal density (arrow) between the anterior and posterior crura of the stapes. Axial CT image one level below (**b**) shows the persistent stapedial artery within a separate bony canal (arrow) overlying the promontory. The foramen spinosum was aplastic (not shown)

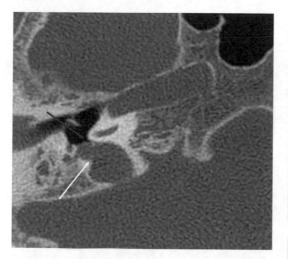

Fig. 4 Axial CT image shows a right jugular bulb with prominent diverticulum (red arrow) which severely narrows the adjacent round window niche, slit like (white arrow)

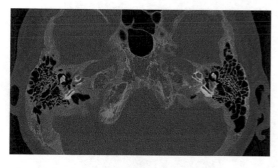

Fig. 5 Elderly male with mixed hearing loss. Axial CT image shows diffuse bone disease (diffuse osteopenia, cortical thickening and coarsening of the trabeculae) involving the temporal bones and the rest of the visualised skull base compatible with Paget's disease

Inner Ear Hearing Loss: Meniere's Disease, Labyrinthitis and Semicircular Canal Dehiscence").

> **Tip**
> - *In the setting of congenital CHL and normal imaging, consider congenital stapedial fixation secondary to failure of differentiation of the lamina stapedialis into annular ligament. This finding cannot be seen on imaging and is confirmed during surgery.*

> **Remember**
> - What do the audiometry and otoscopic findings reveal?
> - Approach the ear from outside to inside; follow the path of sound conduction.
> - Use reconstruction to make subtle asymmetries along the OC more conspicuous.

Further Reading

Chen D, Phillips, CD. Imaging the patient with hearing loss. https://appliedradiology.com/articles/mdct-diagnosis-of-acquired-hearing-loss

Nguyen T, Pulickal G, Singh A, Lingam R (2019) Conductive hearing loss with a "dry middle ear cleft"—a comprehensive pictorial review with CT. Eur J Radiol 110:74–80. https://doi.org/10.1016/j.ejrad.2018.11.024. Epub 2018 Nov 22. Review

Ho ML (2019) Third window lesions. Neuroimaging Clin N Am 29(1):57–92. https://doi.org/10.1016/j.nic.2018.09.005. Review

Imaging Approach to Sensorineural Hearing Loss

Geoiphy George Pulickal

Contents

Abstract

This chapter explains the pathophysiology of sensorineural hearing loss. The various etiologies have been systematically classified, and a stepwise approach on how to tackle the imaging is provided. Detailed checklists of important features will help the reader to pinpoint the relevant pathology for various imaging modalities.

1 What Is Sensorineural Hearing Loss (SNHL)?

SNHL refers to hearing loss attributed to dysfunction of the sensory (cochlea) or neural (retro-cochlear, i.e., vestibulocochlear nerve, nuclei, and the rest of the central auditory pathway) components of hearing. *Audiometry shows increased hearing thresholds without any air-bone gap.* SNHL is more common than CHL, but unfortunately, imaging is often normal.

2 Choice of Imaging

MRI is usually the imaging modality of choice, although CT can be complementary. MRI provides an assessment of the intra-labyrinthine structures, seventh and eight nerve complex, and the cerebellopontine angles. Some lesions such

G. G. Pulickal (✉)
Department of Diagnostic Radiology, Khoo Teck Puat Hospital, Singapore, Singapore
e-mail: pulickal.george.geoiphy@ktph.com.sg

© Springer Nature Switzerland AG 2021
G. G. Pulickal et al. (eds.), *Temporal Bone Imaging Made Easy*,
Medical Radiology Diagnostic Imaging, https://doi.org/10.1007/978-3-030-70635-7_4

as retrofenestral otosclerosis and lesions involving the bony otic capsule are better appreciated on CT.

3   Assessment Pathway

As mentioned earlier, imaging in SNHL may not show any definite causative lesion; thus, it is important to approach the imaging in a systematic manner.

Search for lesions must commence from the cochlea and the vestibulocochlear nerve. Continue onward to assess the region of the cochlear nuclei (dorsal and ventral cochlear nuclei) in the medulla, then follow the course of the lateral lemniscus through the superior olivary nucleus in the pons up to the inferior colliculus of the midbrain, from there the medial geniculate body in the thalamus, and finally on to the superior temporal gyrus (the primary auditory cortex) that lies just beneath the lateral sulcus in the superior aspect of the temporal lobe (Fig. 1).

4   Cochlea (Sensory Component)

Abnormality of cochlea may be microscopic (e.g. at the level of the organ of Corti) and thus blind to imaging or macroscopic. Lesions that distort the configuration of the labyrinth or alter its signal/density would be demonstrated on imaging. Various things to be assessed on CT and MRI are enumerated below.

Fig. 1 Central auditory pathway. (Illustrated by Dr. Somu Victor, Auckland)

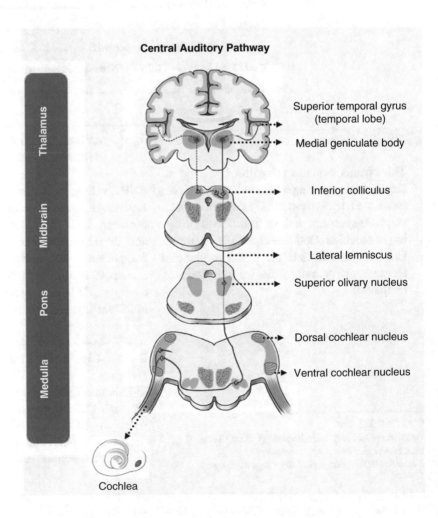

CT	MRI
• Configuration of the cochlea, vestibule, and semicircular canals (any deformity and abnormal enlargement of the vestibular aqueduct?)	• The configuration of the cochlea, vestibule, and semicircular canals (any deformity and abnormal enlargement of the vestibular aqueduct)
• Evaluate for bony replacement of the cochlea, vestibule, or semicircular canals (labyrinthitis ossificans—Fig. 2)	• Loss or attenuation of fluid signal of cochlea, vestibule, or semicircular canals on the T2W sequences (inflammation, hemorrhage, or tumor)
• In the setting of trauma: – Assess for fractures involving the cochlea, vestibule, or semicircular canals – Is there any pneumolabyrinth, it could indicate a peri-lymphatic fistula even if the fracture itself is not visible	• Any post-contrast enhancement of the cochlea, vestibule, or semicircular canals can be due to inflammation/infection or tumor (Fig. 3)
• Search for peri-cochlear lucency (retrofenestral otosclerosis)	• Look for peri-cochlear high T2W signal changes, with or without enhancement (retrofenestral otosclerosis)
• Assess density of the temporal bone (in cases of bony dysplasia)	• Assessment of Meniere's disease requires a special protocol (refer Sect. 4 in chapter "Other causes of Inner Ear Hearing Loss: Meniere's Disease, Labyrinthitis and Semicircular Canal Dehiscence")

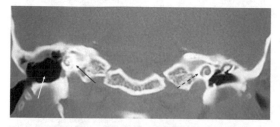

Fig. 2 Coronal CT image shows bony replacement (labyrinthine ossificans) of the right cochlea (red arrow) secondary to inflammation related to cholesteatoma (note the large post-operative mastoid cavity—white arrow). Note the normal left cochlea for comparison (red dashed arrow)

Check List for Cochlea Abnormalities
- **Congenital**: Large vestibular aqueduct, varying degrees of cochlea aplasia, etc.
- **Infective/inflammatory**: Bacterial/viral labyrinthitis, Ramsey-Hunt syndrome, etc.
- **Tumor**: Intracochlea Schwannoma are rare (originating in the Scala tympani)
- **Trauma**: Fractures, penetrating injury, barotrauma, hemorrhage (may be secondary to coagulopathy or labyrinthitis), peri-lymphatic fistula, etc.
- **Miscellaneous**: Meniere's disease, fibrous dysplasia, cochlea otosclerosis, osteogenesis imperfecta, etc.

Tip
- If the membranous labyrinthine enhancement is diffuse, consider inflammatory or infective causes, e.g., Ramsey-Hunt syndrome, tympanogenic labyrinthitis, etc.
- If the enhancement is focal, consider intra-labyrinthine schwannoma, which can arise anywhere along the membranous labyrinth (Fig. 4).

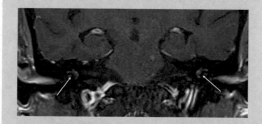

Fig. 3 Coronal post-contrast MRI image shows mild diffuse enhancement of vestibule and semicircular canals bilaterally (arrows); labyrinthitis

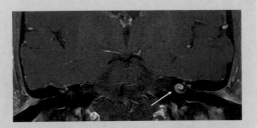

Fig. 4 Coronal post-contrast MRI image shows homogenous intense enhancement confined to the left cochlea (arrow) and sparing the rest of inner ear; labyrinthine Schwannoma

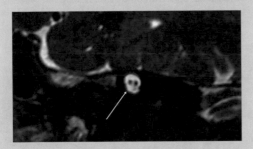

Fig. 5 Patient with long-standing SNHL. Sagittal T2 MR image shows an absent cochlear nerve in the antero-inferior quadrant of the IAC (arrow)

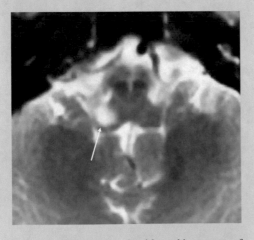

Fig. 6 Patient presented with sudden onset of right-sided SNHL. Axial T2 weighted MR image shows a focal T2 signal prolongation in the right medulla oblangata in the expected location of the right cochlea nuclei, compatible with an acute infarct

5   Cochlea Nerve (Neural Component)

Lesions along the neural pathway are far more common than abnormality within the cochlea itself (sensory component). Unilateral symptoms are usually due to the lesions up to the cochlea nuclei, and lesions beyond this result in bilateral hearing loss. MRI is the best modality of assessment. The following features need to be assessed:

CT	MRI

• The caliber of the cochlear nerve canal. A stenotic canal usually indicate that the cochlear nerve is absent or hypoplastic	• Presence or absence of the cochlear nerve (Fig. 5) on high-resolution heavy T2W sequences
	  – In congenital cochlear nerve hypoplasia, the cochlear nerve is still present but smaller in size
	  – In acquired cochlear nerve atrophy, the cochlear nerve shows decreased signal intensity and an indistinct outline, usually involving the distal segment first

• A widened canal, either diffusely or focally, can be due to tumor, likely an acoustic schwannoma	• Mass lesions in the internal auditory canal and/or cerebellopontine angle; usually acoustic schwannoma or meningioma

• The internal auditory canal can be narrowed by bony dysplasia like fibrous dysplasia, Engelmann's disease, Paget's disease, etc.	• Abnormal enhancement
	  – Of the cochlear nerve itself could be due to neuritis
	  – Meningeal enhancement within the internal auditory canal can be due to meningitis, neurosarcoidosis, Ramsay Hunt's syndrome (the ipsilateral facial and vestibulocochlear nerves might enhance as well)

	• Compression of the cochlear nerve by aneurysm or dolichoectasia (although whether this is incidental or the actual cause of the SHNL is still a subject of much debate)

Check List for Cochlea Nerve Abnormalities
- **Congenital**: Agenesis of the nerve, arachnoid or epidermoid cyst, etc.
- **Infective/inflammatory**: Bacterial/viral neuritis, neurosarcoidosis, leptomeningeal disease, etc.
- **Tumor**: Cerebellopontine angle lesions, i.e., acoustic Schwannoma (most common), meningioma, lipoma, etc.
- **Vascular**: Aneurysms, dolichoectasia (controversial), etc.
- **Miscellaneous**: Atrophy, Engelmann's disease, etc.

Further Reading

Swartz JD (1996) Sensorineural hearing deficit: a systematic approach based on imaging findings. Radiographics 16(3):561–574. Review

Verbist BM (2012) Imaging of sensorineural hearing loss: a pattern-based approach to diseases of the inner ear and cerebellopontine angle. Insights Imaging 3(2):139–153. https://doi.org/10.1007/s13244-011-0134-z. Epub 2011 Dec 9

6 Rest of the Auditory Pathway (Neural Component)

The intra-axial central acoustic pathway should be assessed for lesions such as masses, vascular pathologies such as strokes, bleeds, hemosiderosis, or arteriovenous malformations, and demyelinating plaques (Fig. 6).

Remember
- Imaging in SNHL is often normal.
- Systematically assess the sensory and neural components as described.
- Follow the auditory pathway.
- Enhancement in the labyrinth is always abnormal.

Imaging Approach to Tinnitus

Deepak Bulla and Geoiphy George Pulickal

Contents

Abstract

This chapter explains what tinnitus implies and clarifies often-used terminology. An assessment pathway is formulated, and common causes are classified and enumerated. The rationale for choosing the appropriate imaging modality is explained. A rapid imaging checklist is provided to allow the reader to efficiently assess different anatomical areas to pinpoint pathology.

D. Bulla
Vijaya Diagnostic Center, Hyderabad, India

G. G. Pulickal (✉)
Department of Diagnostic Radiology, Khoo Teck
Puat Hospital, Singapore, Singapore
e-mail: pulickal.george.geoiphy@ktph.com.sg

1   What Is Tinnitus?

Tinnitus is the perception of internal noise in the ears; it can either be pulsatile, when it is in tandem with the patients' pulse, or nonpulsatile (more common). If the sound is exclusively perceived by the patient, it is termed as "subjective," but if an examiner can appreciate the sound as well (usually pulsatile) it is labeled as "objective."

Tinnitus can be the result of a number of health conditions; in many instances, the etiology is away from temporal bone. Imaging is unfortunately often normal in cases of nonpulsatile tinnitus. Imaging is performed to exclude any structural abnormality, which is discussed later in this chapter.

Imaging in pulsatile tinnitus and objective tinnitus tends to reveal some abnormality, usually of a vascular nature (vascular mass or vascular anomaly), although whether these are incidental or causative is often difficult to confirm.

2 Assessment Pathway

Simple external ear canal cerumen can cause tinnitus, but this is usually excluded by clinicians before referring the patient to imaging. On otoscopy, presence of a "vascular tympanic membrane" (red or blue drum) is an indicator of a likely vascular cause and allows focusing on specific vascular/structural abnormalities (refer Sect. 1 in chapter "Common Otoscopic Signs, Imaging of Common Surgeries and Implants").

An anatomical, stepwise approach is recommended to facilitate a thorough search; the most common causes are enumerated below (Table 1).

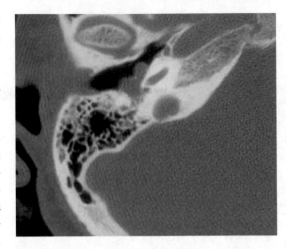

Fig. 1 Axial CT image showing a lobulated soft tissue mass overlying the cochlear promontory, glomus tympanicum

3 Common Causes (Table 1)

Table 1 Common causes of tinnitus

Middle-ear pathology	• Glomus tympanicum (Fig. 1) • Glomus jugulare • Dehiscent or aberrant ICA • Variant jugular bulb anatomy (ectatic, high riding jugular bulb, or jugular diverticulum) (Fig. 2)
Inner-ear pathology	• Vestibular schwannoma • Aberrant vascular loops • Otosclerosis • Meniere's disease
Miscellaneous	• Brain stem pathology (ischemia, demyelination etc.) • Paget's disease • Carotid artery stenosis • Dural venous sinus dehiscence (Fig. 3) • Persistent stapedial artery (look for absent foramen spinosum) • Temporomandibular joint dysfunction • Intracranial hypertension • Vascular malformations of scalp • Eustachian tube dysfunction

> **Tip**
> • *Intra-meatal vascular loops (Fig. 4) (usually the anterior inferior cerebellar artery) are an often observed finding both incidentally and in symptomatic patients, although their significance is highly debatable. When screening for tinnitus, it is recommended to describe this finding.*

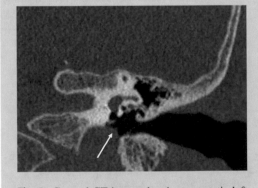

Fig. 2 Coronal CT image showing an ectatic left jugular bulb with dehiscence of the overlying bone, the bulb indents upon the floor of the middle ear cavity (arrow)

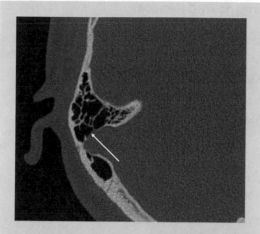

Fig. 3 Axial CT image showing a sigmoid sinus with dehiscence of the overlying bone separating it from the mastoid air cells. This gives rise to the classical "air-on-sinus" sign (arrow)

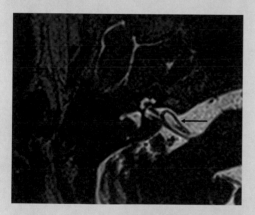

Fig. 4 MR image of a patient with right-sided intermittent tinnitus shows the presence of an intrameatal vascular loop which may or may not be the cause of the symptoms. No other potential causes could be identified

4 Choice of Imaging

Given the diverse nature of possible underlying causes, CT and MRI imaging are complementary, as no imaging modality is perfect in all situations.

Contrast-enhanced CT of the temporal bones is usually the first line of imaging (especially when a "vascular TM" is encountered); it allows for evaluation of the middle ear, aberrant vasculature, and osseous pathology on a single modality. A direct contrast CT is sufficient, and standard high-resolution images should be reconstructed from acquired data to evaluate the ossicular chain and inner ear for subtle abnormalities such as otosclerosis.

Contrast-enhanced MRI study is clearly better in assessing the inner-ear labyrinth, cerebellopontine angles, cisternal, and brain stem pathology. Addition of MRA or MRV helps to delineate possible vascular anomalies as well. If tinnitus presents with associated hearing loss, headache, giddiness, etc., detailed evaluation by MRI should be done.

> **Tip**
> - *If the tinnitus is altered by vascular compression, i.e. augmented or stopped, then a vascular cause is highly likely, and additional angiogram imaging of the neck and brain is imperative.*

5   Quick Imaging Check List

Check List
- Ossicular chain, particularly the stapes footplate—otosclerosis.
- Fenestral and retrofenestral region—demineralized areas—otosclerosis.
- Cochlear   promontory—glomus tympanicum.
- Aberrant or dehiscent ICA canal.
- Anatomical variations or dehiscence of the jugular bulb or dural venous sinuses.
- Cerebellopontine angle space-occupying lesions—vestibular Schwannoma.
- Neurovascular conflict/intra-meatal vascular loops
- Brain stem pathology—ischemia and demyelination
- TMJ pathology—arthritis and synovitis

Suggested Reading

Branstetter BF, Weissman JL (2006) The radiologic evaluation of tinnitus. Eur Radiol 16(12):2792–2802. Epub 2006 May 23

Madani G, Connor SE (2009) Imaging in pulsatile tinnitus. Clin Radiol 64(3):319–328. https://doi.org/10.1016/j.crad.2008.08.014

Vattoth S, Shah R, Curé JK (2010) A compartment-based approach for the imaging evaluation of tinnitus. Am J Neuroradiol 31(2):211–218. https://doi.org/10.3174/ajnr.A1704

Imaging Approach to Otorrhea

Geoiphy George Pulickal

Contents

Abstract

This chapter summarises the potential causes for otorrhea and indications for imaging. A pathway of assessment is formulated in which the key features of otomastoiditis and CSF otorrhea are explained.

1   What Is Otorrhea?

Otorrhea refers to the discharge of fluid from the external ear. The source of otorrhea can be external ear canal, middle ear or cranium.

Otomastoiditis (acute and chronic) accounts for the vast majority of otorrhea along with *otitis externa*. As such, the cause is often clinically obvious and imaging is reserved to determine the extent of disease, screening for possible complications and anatomical variants of surgical importance.

2   Choice of Imaging

Unenhanced CT of temporal bone is an excellent first-line investigation, with further imaging like post-contrast CT or MRI only reserved to answer specific follow-up questions.

3   Assessment Pathway

When dealing with otorrhea, it is important to establish the duration of discharge (whether acute or chronic) and the nature of the discharge (i.e. serous, purulent, or clear).

G. G. Pulickal (✉)
Department of Diagnostic Radiology, Khoo Teck Puat Hospital, Singapore, Singapore
e-mail: pulickal.george.geoiphy@ktph.com.sg

© Springer Nature Switzerland AG 2021
G. G. Pulickal et al. (eds.), *Temporal Bone Imaging Made Easy*,
Medical Radiology Diagnostic Imaging, https://doi.org/10.1007/978-3-030-70635-7_6

Additional information such as associated hearing loss, vertigo, cranial nerve palsies, periauricular/external ear canal inflammation, history of diabetes etc. could indicate possible complications. History of antecedent trauma or instrumentation should prompt suspicion for CSF otorrhea.

4   Acute Otorrhea

Acute otomastoiditis is the most common cause of acute otorrhea and does not warrant routine imaging. Scanning is only required when complications are suspected (refer Sect. 3 in chapter 'Imaging of Otomastoiditis, Acute and Chronic').

In such cases, evaluate for signs of coalescent mastoiditis (i.e. opacification of the mastoid air cells with breakdown of the intervening trabeculae and erosion of mastoid cortices) and any periauricular inflammation/collection or abscess; intracranial spread of disease can occur if treatment is delayed.

If the disease is centred in the EAC and there is involvement of the deep spaces of the neck, particularly in a diabetic patient, consider malignant otitis externa (MOE) (Fig. 1). MOE can be

overlooked by physicians and radiologists alike, if there is a lack of awareness.

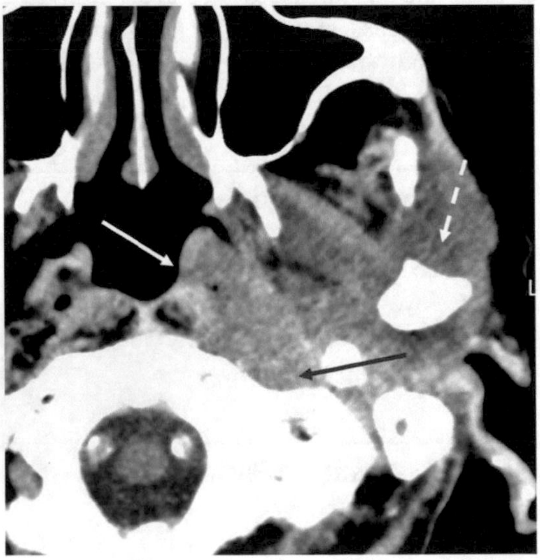

> **Tip**
> • *Acute otomastoiditis with additional symptoms of tinnitus and vertigo are suggestive of inner ear involvement, and cranial nerve palsies raise the possibility of skull base disease. MRI would be needed to assess for intracranial complications.*

5   Chronic Otorrhea

Otomastoiditis is still the most common cause of chronic otorrhea. The temporal bone is usually sclerotic and the middle ear and mastoid air cells opacified (Fig. 2). The aim is to determine whether the opacification is fluid, granulation tissue, cholesteatoma, cholesterol granuloma etc. (refer Sect. 3 in chapter 'Imaging of Otomastoiditis, Acute and Chronic') As in acute otorrhea, exclude any potential complications.

6   CSF Otorrhea

Establish whether the discharge is spontaneous or post-traumatic in nature. Post-traumatic patients usually present with a corroborative history and fracture through the tegmen tympani or mastoideum.

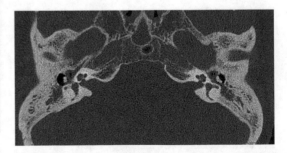

Fig. 1 Axial CT image (soft tissue window) showing malignant otitis externa with involvement of the nasopharynx (white arrow), prevertebral soft tissue (red arrow) and masticator space (white dashed arrow)

Fig. 2 Axial CT image of the temporal bone showing bilateral sclerosed, under-pneumatized and opacified middle ear clefts

In spontaneous CSF otorrhea consider post-surgical, congenital, and acquired causes. Congenital causes are usually related to an abnormal otic capsule (e.g. common cavity, Mondini deformity) and possible fistulous connection to the CSF space.

CSF otorrhea is a known complication of vestibular schwannoma resection and mastoidectomy and can occur weeks after the surgery. It can also be a sequel of erosive disease such as cholesteoma and skull base osteomyelitis.

Evaluate for signs of possible increased intracranial pressure (effacement of the CSF spaces, brain herniation etc.) and defects along the tegmen plate with or without meningo/encephaloceles (requires MRI). If the cause is not readily apparent, then proceed with CSF cisternography (CT or MRI).

Tip
- *Not all discharging clear fluid is CSF; check whether the fluid is indeed CSF by testing positive for beta-transferrin.*

Remember
- Acute or chronic otomastoiditis are the commonest cause of otorrhea.
- In acute setting, rule out complications.
- In chronic otomastoiditis, characterize the middle ear cleft opacification and screen for complications like tympanosclerosis that can be subtle.
- CSF otorrhea may be post-traumatic or spontaneous.

Further Reading

Bardanis J, Batzakakis D, Mamatas S (2003) Types and causes of otorrhea. Auris Nasus Larynx 30(3):253–257 https://www.merckmanuals.com/en-pr/professional/ear,-nose,-and-throat-disorders/approach-to-the-patient-with-ear-problems/otorrhea

Reddy M, Baugnon K (2017) Imaging of cerebrospinal fluid rhinorrhea and otorrhea. Radiol Clin N Am 55(1):167–187. https://doi.org/10.1016/j.rcl.2016.08.005. Review

Imaging Approach to Otalgia

Geoiphy George Pulickal

Contents

Abstract

This chapter explains the types of otalgia and formulates a pathway for detecting potential causes in a systematic manner. A quick checklist for secondary otalgia is provided to help the reader hone in on relevant anatomical areas on the provided imaging.

G. G. Pulickal (✉)
Department of Diagnostic Radiology, Khoo Teck Puat Hospital, Singapore, Singapore
e-mail: pulickal.george.geoiphy@ktph.com.sg

1 What Causes Otalgia?

Otalgia or ear pain can either be primary or secondary. Primary otalgia refers to pain arising from ear pathology itself (e.g. otomastoiditis), and secondary or referred otalgia is ear pain due to causes outside the ear. The cervical plexus, sympathetic fibres and *multiple cranial nerves (V, VII, IX and X)* are responsible for the sensory innervation of the ear. Any pathology in the anatomical structures that share sensory innervation from these cranial nerves could potentially cause ear pain, i.e. nose, paranasal sinuses, oral cavity,

G. G. Pulickal et al. (eds.), *Temporal Bone Imaging Made Easy*,
Medical Radiology Diagnostic Imaging, https://doi.org/10.1007/978-3-030-70635-7_7

pharynx, temporomandibular joint (TMJ), salivary glands etc.

> **Tip**
> - *The trigeminal nerve (CN V) with its rather extensive coverage is the commonest affected pathway, with dental disease and TMJ disorders (Fig. 1) being the most important.*

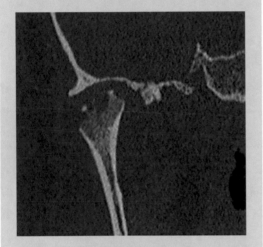

Fig. 1 Coronal CT image shows extensive erosions of the mandibular condyle compatible with arthritis. Secondary otalgia occured via cranial nerve V3

2   Choice of Imaging

CT Temporal bone is the screening imaging of choice and is sufficient in most cases of primary otalgia. MRI is required if intracranial extension is suspected or secondary causes need to be elicited.

> **Tip**
> - *If referred pain is suspected, then include soft tissue window reconstructions and consider widening the extent of the scan to include the salivary glands.*

3   Assessment Pathway

If the ear examination is normal, then consider the causes of referred pain. Try to elicit any history or accompanying clinical signs that could indicate the source of the referred pain, e.g. sinusitis, oral ulcer, poor dental hygiene, jaw stiffness etc.

For analysis of the imaging, it is recommended to follow a systematic approach from outside inwards, starting from the pinna and up to the petrous apex.

3.1   Pinna

Pathology of the pinna such as lacerations, burns or perichondritis (Fig. 2) are readily diagnosed clinically and seldom warrant radiological input.

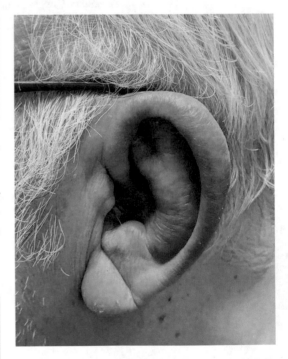

Fig. 2 Otalgia secondary to acute inflammation of the pinna, perichondritis. (Courtesy Dr. Amanda Cheang)

3.2 External Ear Canal (EAC)

Most EAC pathology like foreign bodies, keratosis obturans, acute otitis externa or folliculitis are usually diagnosed clinically and do not need imaging.

Malignant otitis externa is an exception, since its virulent course requires aggressive management, and delineation of disease extent by imaging is necessary. EAC cholesteatoma because of its local erosions would need assessment of extent as well. Squamous cell carcinoma of the EAC is a rare cause and at times difficult to distinguish from cholesteatoma (refer Sect. 2 in chapters "Radiological Features of Otitis Externa" and "Imaging of External Ear Masses: Cholesteatoma and Tumours").

3.3 Middle Ear and Mastoid

Acute otitis media is the most common cause of otalgia, and imaging is usually reserved to exclude complications such as brain abscess, dural venous thrombosis etc. (refer Sect. 3 in chapter "Imaging of Otomastoiditis, Acute and Chronic").

Petrous apex pathology such as apicitis (Gradenigo syndrome), cholesterol granuloma or mucocele are rare causes of ear pain (refer Sect. 5 in chapter "Imaging of the Petrous Apex, Cerebello-Pontine Angles and Jugular Foramen").

4 Secondary Otalgia (Around the Temporal Bone) Checklist

Secondary Otalgia (Around the Temporal Bone) Checklist

- Naso and retropharynx: look out for nasopharyngeal tumours, retropharyngeal lymphadenopathy or abscesses (Fig. 3)
- Oral cavity and oropharynx: tumours of the tongue or tonsils, dental disease (caries, periodontal disease, impacted teeth etc.), tonsillitis and its complications (Fig. 4)
- Paranasal sinus: sinusitis, tumours and even deviated nasal septum (Fig. 5)
- TMJ: mal-positioning, degeneration or disc disease
  - Parotid gland; parotitis, ductal obstruction, neoplasms (Fig. 6)

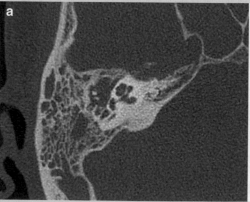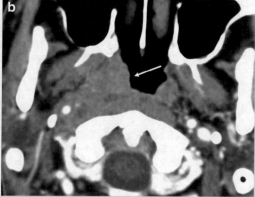

Fig. 3 (**a** and **b**) CT axial image of a patient with right-sided otalgia shows a completely opacified middle ear cleft (**a**). Caudal axial image in soft tissue window (**b**) shows a right-sided nasopharyngeal mass as the underlying cause (arrow)

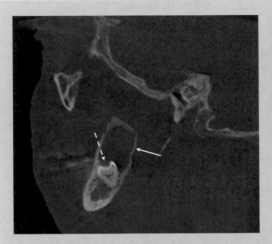

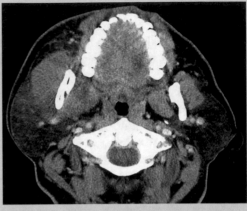

Fig. 4 Cone-beam CT sagittal image of a patient with right-sided otalgia shows a large dentigerous cyst involving the body of the mandible (arrow) secondary to an unerupted third molar tooth (dashed arrow)

Fig. 6 Axial CT image of a patient with right-sided otalgia shows gross inflammation of the right side of the face secondary to parotiditis, note the secondary involvement of the adjacent right masticator space

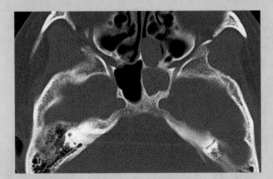

Fig. 5 Axial CT image of a patient with otalgia shows chronic inflammation of the left sphenoid sinus secondary to an obstructed polyp at the left sphenoethmoidal recess. Pathway of referred pain is through cranial nerve VII via the posterior auricular nerve

Suggested Reading

Chen RC, Khorsandi AS, Shatzkes DR, Holliday RA (2009) The radiology of referred otalgia. AJNR Am J Neuroradiol 30(10):1817–1823. https://doi.org/10.3174/ajnr.A1605. Epub 2009 Oct 1. Review

Weissman JL (1997) A pain in the ear: the radiology of otalgia. AJNR Am J Neuroradiol 18(9):1641–1651

Clinical Otoscopy Findings and Imaging of Common Surgeries and Implants

Ya Fang Amanda Cheang and Seng Beng Yeo

Contents

Y. F. A. Cheang (✉)
Department of Otorhinolaryngology,
Woodlands Health Campus, Singapore, Singapore
e-mail: amanda_cheang@whc.sg

S. B. Yeo
Department of Otorhinolaryngology,
Tan Tock Seng Hospital, Singapore, Singapore
e-mail: seng_beng_yeo@ttsh.com.sg

Abstract

A basic understanding of otoscopic signs and common otological surgeries is necessary in order to provide surgeons with a relevant report. This chapter explains common otoscopic findings and their possible causes. A brief explanation of common otological surgeries and their indications, as well as important anatomical landmarks is provided in a concise manner.

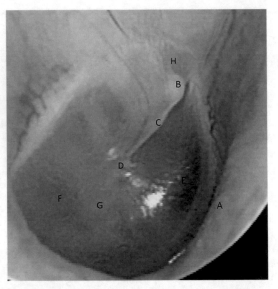

Fig. 1 Otoscopic image of the right tympanic membrane. (A) Bulge of anterior external auditory canal wall. (B) Lateral process of malleus. (C) Handle of malleus. (D) Umbo. (E) Shadow of Eustachian tube opening. (F) Shadow of round window niche. (G) Promontory. (H) Pars flaccida

1 What Is Otoscopy?

Otoscopy is a visual examination of the external auditory canal (EAC), tympanic membrane (TM), and middle ear using a handheld otoscope or microscope.

Under normal conditions, otoscopy allows for only limited inspection of the middle ear through the intact TM (Fig. 1). Classical abnormal otoscopic findings mentioned in the imaging request/history may provide the diagnosis itself or at least narrows the differentials considerably (Tables 1 and 2).

1.1 Otoscopy Features of Common External Auditory Canal (EAC) Conditions

Table 1 Otoscopic Features of Common Conditions of the EAC

EAC Conditions		Otoscopic Findings
(A)	Impacted cerumen	Excessive buildup of cerumen in the EAC
(B)	Keratosis Obturans	Plug of keratin with layered (onion skin) organization associated with a circumferentially widened EAC. May be bilateral
(C)	EAC cholesteatoma	Focal erosion of the EAC wall with squames. Usually unilateral (Fig. 2)
(D)	Acute otitis externa	Erythema and swelling of the EAC skin with purulent debris. Fungal spores may be present
(E)	Malignant otitis externa	Osteomyelitis of the skull base, which may present with inflammatory polyp or granulation, classically arising from the anterior–inferior aspect of the EAC at the osseocartilaginous junction
(F)	Medial canal fibrosis	Stenosis of the medial EAC, usually with discharge. Progression of fibrosis may eventually lead to the appearance of a false fundus and abnormally shallow or blind-ending EAC
(G)	Exostosis	Bony mounds at the anterior and posterior EAC walls, usually bilateral
(H)	Osteoma	Solitary, pedunculated bony mass arising from the tympano-squamous suture line. Usually unilateral
(I)	Malignant tumors	Variable appearance. May be sessile and infiltrative or pedunculated. Ulceration and contact bleeding may be present

1.2 Otoscopy Features of Common Conditions of the Tympanic Membrane and Middle Ear

Table 2 Otoscopic Features of Common Conditions of the Tympanic Membrane (TM) and Middle Ear

TM and Middle Ear Conditions	Otoscopic findings
(A) Chronic suppurative otitis media	Chronic tympanic membrane perforation of the pars tensa with discharge. Discharge may be persistent or intermittent (Fig. 3)
(B) Acquired cholesteatoma	Retraction pocket in the attic or posterior–superior quadrant of the tympanic membrane with accumulation of squamous debris within. Surrounding bony erosion and granulation tissue may be present adjacent to the cholesteatoma (Fig. 4)
(C) Congenital cholesteatoma	Pearly, white lesion in the anterior–superior quadrant of the middle ear behind a normal, intact tympanic membrane
(D) Tympanosclerosis	White plaques on the tympanic membrane

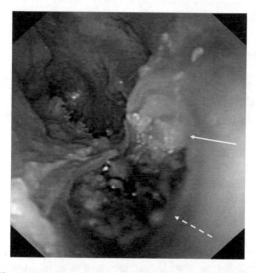

Fig. 2 Otoscopic image of the left EAC showing bony erosion (dashed arrow) in the posteroinferior wall containing squames (arrow), consistent with EAC cholesteatoma

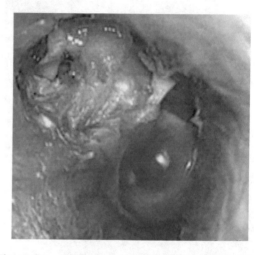

Fig. 4 Otoscopic image of the right medial EAC showing squames within a retracted pars flaccida region of the tympanic membrane and erosion of the surrounding bone, consistent with cholesteatoma

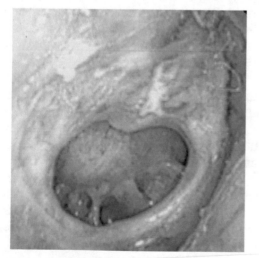

Fig. 3 Otoscopic image of the right medial EAC showing a large central perforation of the tympanic membrane, consistent with chronic suppurative otitis media

1.3 The "Blue Drum" Vs. "Red Mass"

In the presence of an intact tympanic membrane, lesions within the middle ear may not be visualized clearly on otoscopic examination. Certain features such as the color of the lesion may help to narrow down the differentials. Often encountered descriptions such as "blue drum and "red mass" can have a variety of causes, the most common ones being enumerated subsequently (Table 3).

Table 3 Differential Diagnoses of Middle Ear Conditions presenting with a "Blue Drum" or "Red Mass behind the Ear Drum"

Differentials for a "Blue drum"	Differentials for "Red mass behind the ear drum"
• Otitis media with effusion	• Acute otitis media – Inflamed, hyperemic and bulging drum, with pus in the middle ear

• Hemotympanum (Fig. 5)	• Paraganglioma
	  – Glomus tympanicum (centred on promontory (Fig. 6)
	  – Glomus jugulare

• High riding or dehiscent jugular bulb	• Aberrant carotid artery, persistent stapedial artery
• Cholesterol granuloma	• Schwartze sign in Otosclerosis – Red hue over the promontory due to increased vascularity during the otospongiotic phase

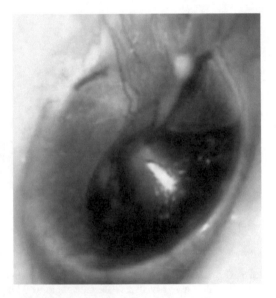

Fig. 5 Otoscopic image of a blue drum due to hemotympanum

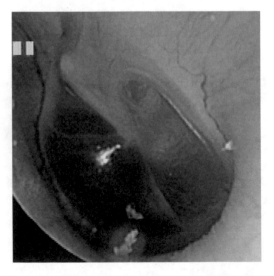

Fig. 6 Otoscopic image of a red mass behind the eardrum due to a glomus tympanicum

2 Common Surgeries

2.1 Tympanoplasty

Tympanoplasty refers to reconstruction of the tympanic membrane and/or ossicular chain. Myringoplasty is a subtype of tympanoplasty involving only reconstruction of the tympanic membrane without attempt at reconstruction of the ossicular chain and prior imaging is rarely required.

2.2 Mastoidectomy

Mastoidectomies are generally performed as curative surgery for cholesteatoma or as a surgical approach for other surgeries, e.g., cochlear implantation and translabyrinthine approach surgery. Pre-operative CT scan is particularly useful in cholesteatoma surgery to assess the extent of disease and presence of complications such as labyrinthine fistula or tegmen erosion. The main types of mastoidectomies include:

Intact canal wall (canal wall up)—Mastoid air cells are removed, but the bony posterior wall of the external auditory canal is kept intact (e.g. cortical mastoidectomy, posterior tympanotomy) (Fig. 7). A well-pneumatized mastoid is better suited for canal wall-up mastoidectomy.

Canal wall down—Mastoid air cells are removed together with the posterior wall of the external auditory canal (Fig. 8). A sclerotic mastoid is better suited for this surgery if performed in a front-to-back fashion.

– Radical mastoidectomy: Canal wall down exteriorization of the middle ear without pres-

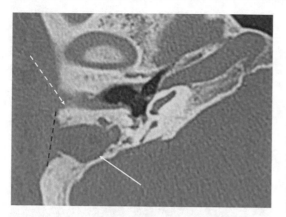

Fig. 7 Axial CT image showing prior "canal-wall up" mastoidectomy with exenteration of the mastoid air cells, removal of the overlying cortex (red dotted line), and preservation of the EAC posterior wall (white dashed arrow). The resultant mastoid cavity is opacified (white arrow) and suspicious for recurrent disease

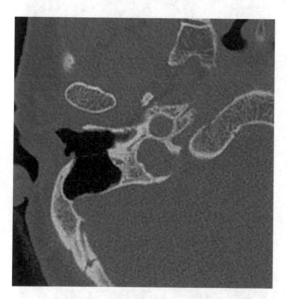

Fig. 8 Axial CT image showing "canal-wall down" mastoidectomy with exenteration of the mastoid air cells and removal of the posterior wall of the EAC (red dotted line)

2.3 Translabyrinthine Approach

This surgery is performed to gain access to tumors or lesions of the internal auditory canal (IAC) and/or cerebellopontine angle (CPA). An MRI scan is the imaging of choice to identify classical characteristics of the primary lesion and its extent. A CT scan can be performed to assess for factors that may restrict accessibility to the IAC, including a low-lying tegmen, anteriorly positioned sigmoid sinus, or high-riding jugular bulb, and to assess for degree of mastoid pneumatization.

> **For all Ear Surgeries: Imaging Findings of General Importance**
> - Low-lying or dehiscent tegmen tympani/mastoideum
> - Anteriorly or laterally positioned sigmoid sinus
> - High-riding and/or large jugular bulb
> - Aberrant carotid artery
> - Large mastoid emissary veins
> - Degree of mastoid pneumatization
> - Aberrant facial nerve anatomy

3 Otological Surgeries Involving Implants

3.1 Ossiculoplasty

Ossiculoplasty refers to the surgical reconstruction of the middle ear conduction pathway to allow sound transmission from tympanic membrane to the oval window.

It is indicated in conductive hearing loss due to ossicular chain discontinuity (e.g. traumatic disruption, erosion secondary to cholesteatoma or CSOM) or fixation (e.g. congenital, post-inflammatory). Regardless of the imaging findings, confirmation of diagnosis is made during surgery by direct visualization and palpation of the ossicles to ascertain fixation or discontinuity as the actual cause.

ervation of the middle ear space. No tympanic membrane graft is placed, thus leaving the middle ear open. The middle ear mucosa is stripped, and the Eustachian tube is plugged (now an obsolete surgery).
- Modified radical mastoidectomy: Canal wall down mastoidectomy with preservation of the middle ear space by performing a tympanoplasty.

Different types of materials can be used to perform an ossiculoplasty. These include autologus grafts (e.g. when the native incus is used as an interposition graft) and alloplastic/synthetic prostheses.

A *Partial ossicular replacement prosthesis (PORP)* connects the tympanic membrane to the capitulum (head) of the stapes in the presence of an intact stapes superstructure and mobile stapes footplate. A *Total ossicular replacement prosthesis (TORP)* connects the tympanic membrane to a mobile stapes footplate in the absence of a stapes superstructure. Success of surgery is determined based on improvement or resolution of conductive hearing loss on post-operative audiogram and post-operative imaging is not routinely performed.

3.2 Stapedectomy and Stapedotomy

These procedures are indicated in conductive hearing loss secondary to fixation of the stapes footplate. The causes include otosclerosis (most commonly), osteogenesis imperfecta, and congenital absence of the oval window. CT scan is useful to identify classical radiological features of otosclerosis, as well as to exclude other potential causes of conductive hearing loss such as malleus head fixation, calcified anterior malleal ligament and superior semicircular canal dehiscence. Regardless of imaging findings, the diagnosis can only be ascertained when the footplate is palpated intra-operatively and confirmed to be immobile.

Stapedectomy refers to the removal of the stapes superstructure and part or whole of the stapes footplate with insertion of a prosthesis through the oval window. *Stapedotomy* involves the removal of the stapes superstructure and creation of a small fenestration in the footplate through which a prosthesis is inserted. Success of surgery is determined by improvement or resolution of conductive hearing loss on post-operative audiogram. Post-operative imaging is not routinely performed. In patients who present with interval recurrence of conductive hearing loss or new sensorineural hearing loss with vestibular symptoms following prior stapes surgery, imaging is performed to look for prosthesis displacement (Figs. 9 and 10) and other complications such as reparative granuloma and perilymphatic fistula.

Tip
Features to look out for on imaging done for patients presenting with vestibular symptoms and/or sensorineural hearing loss following stapes surgery:
– *Overly long prosthesis (look for excessive protrusion of prosthesis into the vestibule)*
– *Perilymphatic fistula (look for pneumolabyrinth and/or middle ear fluid)*
– *Reparative granuloma (look for localized soft tissue mass around the oval window and prosthesis)*

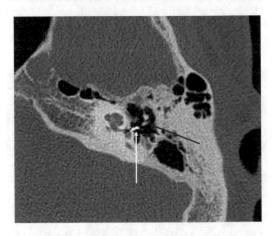

Fig. 9 Axial CT image of a patient with recurrence of conductive hearing loss post stapedotomy, showing dislodgement of the prosthesis (white arrow) off the incus (red arrow)

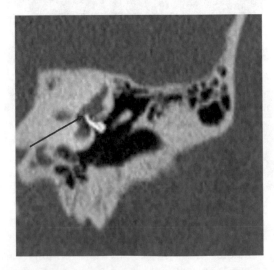

Fig. 10 Coronal CT image of a patient with vertigo post-stapes surgery, showing medial displacement of the prosthesis (red arrow) into the vestibule through the oval window

3.3 Cochlear Implant Surgery

The cochlear implant is an electronic device that converts mechanical sound energy into electrical signals that are transmitted via an electrode array to the inner ear. This electrode array is surgically inserted into the cochlea (via the round window or a cochleostomy) and stimulates the spiral ganglion cells directly.

Indications for surgery include bilateral severe to profound sensorineural hearing loss and selected cases of single-sided severe to profound sensorineural hearing loss.

Key steps involved for electrode insertion are cortical mastoidectomy to identify the mastoid antrum and visualization and access to the round window via a posterior tympanotomy (this involves drilling out a window bounded by the

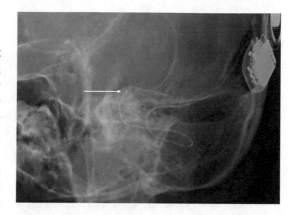

Fig. 11 Modified Stenver's radiograph showing a cochlear implant with malpositioned electrode in the superior semicircular canal

vertical segment of the facial nerve, chorda tympani, and fossa incudis to access the middle ear).

Post-cochlear implant imaging is performed mainly to confirm the position of the electrode array. The most commonly performed view is the Modified Stenver's radiograph (Fig. 11).

Imaging Checklist Prior to Cochlear Implant Insertion

- Assess the degree of mastoid bone pneumatization
- Check for middle ear adhesions and patency of the round window niche
- Exclude labyrinthitis ossificans. Absence of a fluid-filled cochlear duct may indicate fibrosis and could be a precursor to cochlear ossification (on MRI)
- Assess any cochlear abnormalities, e.g., incomplete partition and common cavity, which may influence the choice of electrode. Cochlear and cochlear nerve aplasia (on MRI) are absolute contraindications for cochlear implantation.
- Look for aberrant facial nerve anatomy or anteriorly positioned vertical facial nerve that may restrict the size of the posterior tympanotomy and limit the access for electrode insertion.
- Check for an enlarged vestibular or cochlear aqueduct that may predispose to a perilymph gusher.
- Assess for factors that may necessitate a transection and blind-sac closure of the EAC (e.g. osteoradionecrosis of the temporal bone)

What to Look Out for on the Modified Stenver's View Radiograph

- In general, presence of at least 270° insertion depth angle of the electrode within the cochlea is indicative of a complete insertion in a normal cochlea. (Of note, the optimal insertion depth angle varies depending on the length and design of the electrode used.)
- Electrode array complications such as kinking or tip fold-over.
- Extra-cochlear array misplacement, particularly in anatomically abnormal inner ears.

Post-implant cross-sectional imaging (conventional or cone-beam CT) with multiplanar reconstruction is generally reserved for cases in which the plain radiograph is abnormal or inadequate. Cone-beam CT has the added capability of discerning whether the electrode array is successfully positioned in the Scala tympani or has translocated into the Scala vestibuli/Scala media.

Since intimate knowledge of the inserted device is necessary to reliably report these findings, close collaboration with the surgeon is vital.

3.4   Bone Conduction Implants

A bone conduction implant transfers sound as vibrations into the skull bone and then the inner ear via an audio processor-driven transducer. This transducer is connected to an implantable osseointegrated titanium screw or a floating mass transducer.

It is usually indicated in cases of single-sided deafness, conductive hearing loss and certain cases of mixed hearing loss.

Apart from assessing the cause of the conductive hearing loss and whether it can be surgically corrected, CT scan is also useful to assess the status of the bone in the post-aural region to determine suitability for implant insertion. Presence of osteoradionecrosis may affect the ability of the implant to osseointegrate. In post-mastoidectomy cases, it is important to assess the adequacy of bony surface area available to accomodate the implant. As such, it is useful to report any undue thinning or bony defects in the post-auricular region.

Further Reading

Brackmann DE, Shelton C, Arriaga MA (2016) Otologic surgery, 4th edn. Elsevier, Philadelphia
Connor SEJ (2018) Contemporary imaging of auditory implants. Clin Radiol 73(1):19–34. https://doi.org/10.1016/j.crad.2017.03.002. Epub 2017 Apr 5
Stone JA, Mukherji SK, Jewett BS, Carrasco VN, Castillo M (2000) CT evaluation of prosthetic ossicular reconstruction procedures: what the otologist needs to know. Radiographics 20(3):593–605

Part II

Imaging of External Ear; Pathology

Radiological Features of Otitis Externa

Vincent Ern Yao Chan
and Geoiphy George Pulickal

Contents

Abstract

This chapter discusses the salient features for otitis externa and malignant otitis externa (MOE) and the rationale for available imaging options. The important imaging features and management of MOE are discussed with specific attention being made on how to differentiate this condition from other possible mimics.

V. E. Y. Chan
Department of Diagnostic Imaging, National University Hospital, Singapore, Singapore

G. G. Pulickal (✉)
Department of Diagnostic Radiology, Khoo Teck Puat Hospital, Singapore, Singapore
e-mail: pulickal.george.geoiphy@ktph.com.sg

1 What Is Otitis Externa?

Simply put, otitis externa refers to the inflammation of the external ear, usually just the external ear canal but the pinna can be involved as well.

It is a common problem in humid conditions, among swimmers (also known as swimmer's ear) and users of hearing aids among others. It is readily treated by topical antibiotics and aural toilet, thus rarely requires imaging.

Imaging is reserved in cases of suspected malignant otitis externa (MOE) also known as necrotising external otitis, which could lead to skull base osteomyelitis.

2 Malignant Otitis Externa (MOE)

MOE is a severe, potentially life-threatening infection of the EAC with the potential for rapid involvement of the surrounding soft tissues and skull base.

2.1 Clinical Features and Management

It is usually seen in elderly diabetic or immuno-compromised patients. Patients present with disproportionate symptoms (persistent otalgia and purulent otorrhoea) and non-responsiveness to conventional treatment. Sometimes the presenting symptoms may be nonspecific (e.g. headache, stroke-like symptoms) or even 'silent'. *Pseudomonas aeruginosa* is involved in a high percentage of cases (50–90%). *Cranial nerve deficits* should raise the concern for underlying skull base osteomyelitis (with the facial nerve being the most commonly involved).

Hallmarks of management are early detection, diabetic control, debridement and antibiotic therapy. Imaging is vital to determine the extent of inflammatory spread and localising any possible drainable collection (refer Box: Pathways of Inflammatory Spread).

2.2 Choice of Imaging

Contrast-enhanced MRI (with DWI sequence) of the temporal bone and neck is the preferred imaging modality for diagnosis and follow-up.

CT of the temporal bone (with contrast-enhanced scan of the neck) is another option, since CT is extremely useful for evaluating bone erosion and demineralisation. Use of intravenous contrast is important for evaluation of soft tis-

sues, potential collections and the dural venous sinuses. Ga-67-citrate scans may be used for evaluation of treatment response.

2.3 Imaging Features

Diagnosing MOE when patients present with typical symptoms and clinical signs is usually not a diagnostic challenge. The classical radiological features comprise extensive soft tissue swelling in and around the EAC, as well as bony erosions with or without phlegmon/abscess (Fig. 1).

The real diagnostic challenge arises when clinical symptoms are non-specific and other conditions mimic MOE, i.e. nasopharyngeal carcinoma (NPC), squamous cell carcinoma (SCC) or mastoiditis. The clinical setting, i.e. absence of raised inflammatory markers and different patient profiles (younger and immunocompetent) can help in differentiating MOE from other conditions.

MOE is often incidentally noticed in routine initial imaging (usually a CT scan of the brain) in cases with atypical clinical presentation (mimicking stroke or other intracranial pathology). In such cases, the abnormality is often a 'mass' in the nasopharyngeal region with destructive changes in the skull base detected on the last few slices of the scan and often erroneously diagnosed as NPC (as this is the most common cause in our region – Southeast Asia).

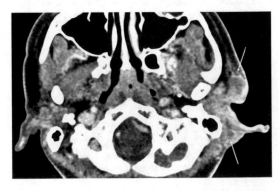

Fig. 1 Contrast-enhanced axial CT image shows florid soft tissue swelling around the left external ear canal with foci of rim enhancing collections (arrows), compatible with MOE. The contralateral side provides excellent comparison

Pathways of Inflammatory Spread

Anterior:

- Involvement of the masticator and parotid spaces

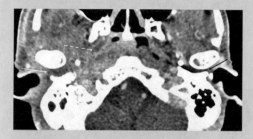

Fig. 2 Contrast-enhanced axial CT image shows severe right-sided MOE with effacement of the retromandibular fat and widening of the TMJ (white arrow). Note the normal contralateral side (black arrow). The inflammation has advanced to involve the prevertebral space along the clivus and nasopharyngeal space (dashed arrow)

- Subtle effacement of the retromandibular fat and widening of the TMJ (Fig. 2)

Medial/contralateral:

- Involvement of the parapharyngeal space (Fig. 2)
- Differentiate from NPC

Posterior:

- Involvement of the mastoid segment of the temporal bone (Fig. 3)
- Differentiate from mastoiditis

Cranial:

- Assess for involvement of the dura, dural venous sinuses, jugular vein and ICA (thrombosis)

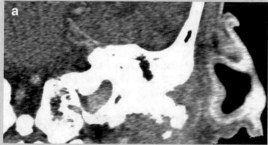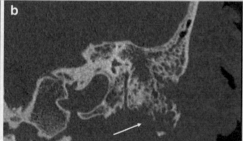

Fig. 3 (a and b) Coronal CT images in soft tissue (a) and bone windows (b) shows extension of the MOE soft tissue inflammation over the mastoid segment, with resultant underlying bony erosions (arrow)

3   MOE versus NPC

Erroneously diagnosing NPC over MOE can often lead to unnecessary biopsies and treatment delays. Both conditions could have overlapping imaging features, i.e. nasopharyngeal mass with skull base destruction, marrow replacement, etc. Note the differentiating features summarised subsequently (Table 1) (Figs. 4 and 5).

Table 1 Malignant otitis externa versus nasopharyngeal carcinoma

Malignant otitis externa	Nasopharyngeal carcinoma
Presence of abscesses (rim enhancement and focal restricted diffusion)	Abscesses are not a typical feature
Diffuse soft tissue inflammation (facilitated diffusion on DWI/ADC) with preservation of normal soft tissue architecture	Mass distorts the adjacent soft tissue/musculature and shows restricted diffusion with low ADC values
Diffuse hyperintense T2WI signal	Hypo to iso-intense signal on T2WI
"Mass" surface tends to be smooth	Mass surface tends to be more irregular
Lymphadenopathy is not prominent (peri-auricular if at all)	Prominent lymphadenopathy (cervical, posterior and retropharyngeal)
Involvement of lateral structures (i.e. masticator and parotid spaces)	Cranio-caudal extension is more likely

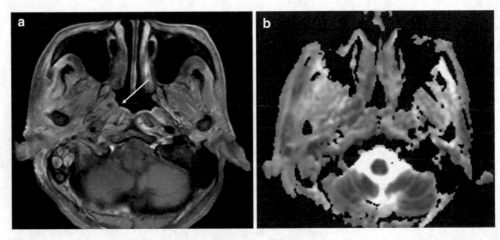

Fig. 4 (**a** and **b**) Post-contrast axial (**a**) and DWI ADC (**b**) images of patient with right-sided MOE. Extensive soft tissue inflammation centred upon the right EAC with extension to the lateral pharyngeal recess (arrow), note the preservation of the underlying architecture and facilitated diffusion on the corresponding ADC image

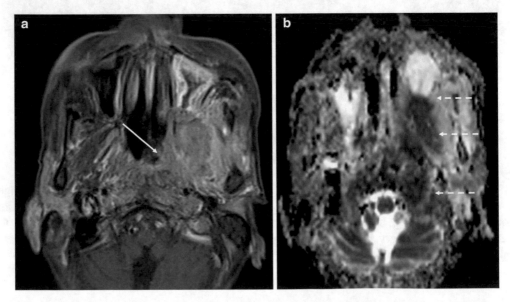

Fig. 5 (**a** and **b**) Post-contrast axial (**a**) and DWI ADC (**b**) images of patient with left-sided nasopharyngeal carcinoma. Irregular soft tissue mass centred upon the left lateral pharyngeal recess (arrow) with distortion of the underlying architecture and restricted diffusion on the corresponding ADC image (dashed arrows). Note the lack of superficial soft tissue inflammation around the external ear

4 MOE versus SCC

Squamous cell carcinoma of the external ear canal can have a strikingly similar appearance to MOE in terms of soft tissue involvement, direction of spread and underlying bony destruction (with the TMJ being frequently involved) (Fig. 6).

The cohort of patients differs from MOE in being slightly younger (although the age range can be wide), immunocompetent and aseptic. On imaging, SCC tends to distort the soft tissue architecture, T2WI hyperintensity of the lesion is markedly lower (than on MOE), the lesion shows restricted diffusion (vs facilitated diffusion on MOE, barring focal abscesses) and accompanying (metastatic) lymphadenopathy is more pronounced than with MOE (small volume reactive nodes) (Fig. 7).

> **Tip**
> - *Care must be made to differentiate tumour necrosis from loculated collection/abscesses.*

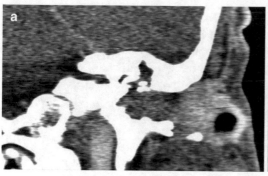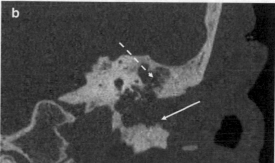

Fig. 6 (**a** and **b**) Coronal CT images in soft tissue (**a**) and bone windows (**b**) of a patient with confirmed squamous cell carcinoma of the left ear. Note the extensive soft tissue thickening in and around the EAC with opacification of the middle ear. There are associated erosions of the bony canal (arrow) and periosteal reaction in the epitympanum (dashed arrow)

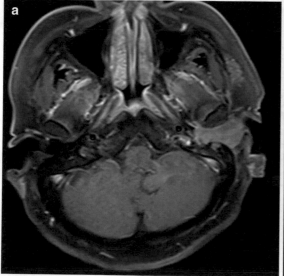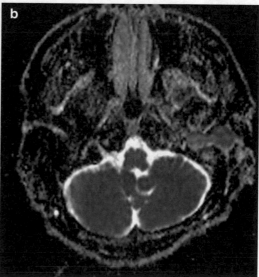

Fig. 7 (**a** and **b**) Axial post-contrast (**a**) and DWI ADC (**b**) images of a patient with left-sided EAC squamous cell carcinoma. Note the enhancing soft tissue mass filling the left EAC and middle ear, which shows restricted diffusion on the corresponding ADC image

5 MOE versus Mastoiditis

Mastoiditis refers to inflammation of the mastoid segment of the temporal bone, i.e. the mastoid air cells. When present along with otitis media (which it invariably is), then it is referred to as otomastoiditis. It can give rise to multiple complications such as subperiosteal and Bezold abscesses, bone disease (coalescent mastoiditis) etc. (Fig. 8). Imaging is required in cases of mastoiditis if complications are suspected.

In severe cases of mastoiditis, the inflammation can extend anteriorly to involve the EAC and can mimic MOE. However, in mastoiditis, the epicentre of inflammation is more posterior; opacification of the mastoid air cells and erosions of the intervening septae (coalescence) dominate over inflammation in the more anterior and medial spaces.

Essentially, mastoiditis is an inflammation of the bone that may have secondary surrounding soft tissue extensions, while MOE is predominantly a soft tissue inflammation with possible underlying bony involvement. Mastoiditis is treated markedly differently from MOE with intravenous antibiotics, tympanostomy tube placement and, if necessary, mastoidectomy.

> **What the Surgeon Wants to Know**
> 1. Extent of disease and associated complications, e.g. skull base osteomyelitis, venous sinus thrombosis, etc.
> 2. Any drainable abscesses; if yes, where exactly and how large?
> 3. Is there bilateral ear involvement? (poorer prognosis)
> 4. Any other diagnosis with differing management? (NPC, SCC or mastoiditis?)

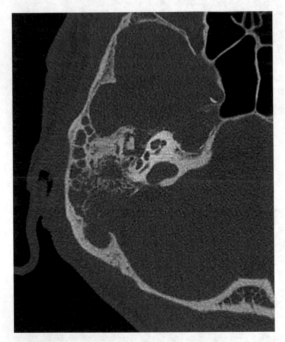

Fig. 8 Axial CT image of patient with severe right-sided mastoiditis shows complete opacification of the right middle ear and mastoid air cells along with erosions of the intervening bony septae. Note the distinct lack of overlying soft tissue thickening

Further Reading

Adams A, Offiah C (2012) Central skull base osteomyelitis as a complication of necrotizing otitis externa: imaging findings, complications, and challenges of diagnosis. Clin Radiol 67(10):e7–e16

Goh JPN, Karandikar A, Loke SC, Tan TY (2017) Skull base osteomyelitis secondary to malignant otitis externa mimicking advanced nasopharyngeal cancer: MR imaging features at initial presentation. Am J Otolaryngol 38(4):466–471. https://doi.org/10.1016/j.amjoto.2017.04.007.

van Kroonenburgh AM, van der Meer WL, Bothof RJ, van Tilburg M, van Tongeren J, Postma AA (2018) Advanced imaging techniques in skull base osteomyelitis due to malignant otitis externa. Curr Radiol Rep 6(1):3

Imaging of External Ear Canal Masses: Cholesteatoma and Tumours

Vincent Ern Yao Chan
and Geoiphy George Pulickal

Contents

Abstract

This chapter explains the clinical and imaging features of external auditory canal cholesteatoma. Detailed discussions on how to differentiate cholesteatoma from osteoradionecrosis, keratosis obturans and medial canal fibrosis are provided. The chapter then goes on to discuss malignancy of the EAC with a dedicated attention being made to address the specific concerns of the referring surgeons. Finally, a quick tabular reference is given for easy summary of all soft tissue lesions affecting the EAC.

V. E. Y. Chan
Department of Diagnostic Imaging, National
University Hospital, Singapore, Singapore

G. G. Pulickal (✉)
Department of Diagnostic Radiology, Khoo Teck
Puat Hospital, Singapore, Singapore
e-mail: pulickal.george.geoiphy@ktph.com.sg

© Springer Nature Switzerland AG 2021
G. G. Pulickal et al. (eds.), *Temporal Bone Imaging Made Easy*,
Medical Radiology Diagnostic Imaging, https://doi.org/10.1007/978-3-030-70635-7_10

1 External Auditory Canal Cholesteatoma (EACC)

1.1 What Is an EACC?

Non-neoplastic lesion of the temporal bone lined by keratinizing stratified squamous epithelium with surrounding periostitis and bone erosion. EAC cholesteatoma is uncommon and occurs either spontaneously or after instrumentation/trauma.

1.2 Clinical Features and Management

Middle-aged (fourth to seventh decades) patients present with otorrhea and otalgia (less commonly conductive hearing loss (CHL)). Otoscopic findings of squames with bony erosion make the diagnosis often straightforward.

Aural toilet and debridement are the hallmarks of treatment with more extensive surgery like canaloplasty and mastoidectomy rarely being required. Unfortunately, recurrence is a common problem in larger lesions.

1.3 Choice of Imaging and Imaging Features

Non-contrast high-resolution CT of temporal bone is the imaging technique of choice. MR imaging provides complementary information (e.g. restricted diffusion) but is rarely needed (Fig. 1).

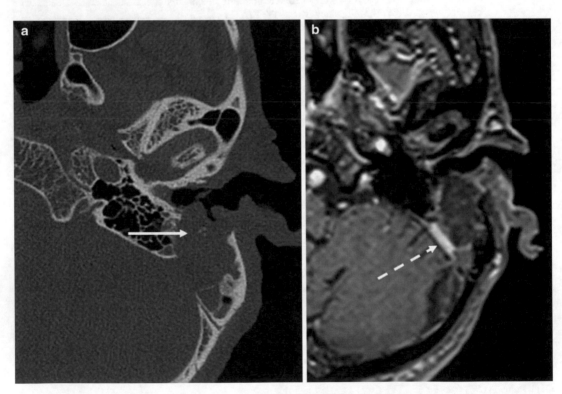

Fig. 1 (**a** and **b**) Axial CT image (**a**) of a patient with known EACC shows a large infiltrative soft tissue mass eroding through the posterior wall of the EAC into the underlying mastoid segment of the temporal bone and possibly involving the sigmoid sinus, note the intramural bone fragments (arrow). Corresponding post-contrast axial MR image (**b**) confirms destruction of the sigmoid plate and mass effect upon the underlying sinus (dashed arrow), but normal contrast opacification of the sinus is preserved

> **Tip**
> - *Lack of intramural bone fragments does not exclude EACC.*
> - *The otoscopic presence of squames in the EAC is probably the most important clinical finding that would point to the disease, even in the absence of classical radiological findings.*

The classical appearance is that of a unilateral discrete soft tissue mass in the EAC with underlying bony erosions and intramural bone fragments (seen~50%) (Fig. 1). Erosions tend to involve the posterior or inferior walls and can be smooth or irregular depending on the degree of associated periostitis and necrosis (Fig. 2).

1.4 Differentials

Clinically, osteo-radionecrosis (ORN) can also present with squames and bony erosion/fragmentation and might pose a diagnostic challenge. Radiologically, EAC cholesteatoma needs to be differentiated from keratosis obturans, medial canal fibrosis, malignancy and MOE (refer Sect. 2 in chapter 'Radiological Features of Otitis Externa'). Some normal variants like the foramen of Huschke (also known as the foramen tympani-cum) (Fig. 3) should not pose a serious diagnostic dilemma.

(a) **ORN** is a delayed complication of prior head and neck radiotherapy, the temporal bone being particularly susceptible due to its relatively poor vascularity. It prominently involves the mastoid air cells with disruption of air cell septation on a background of radiation-induced otomastoiditis. Imaging wise, ORN presents with bony changes of osteopaenia, fragmentation and coarsening of the trabecular architecture without any associated soft tissue mass (in fact a thinning of the overlying soft tissue is often noticed) (Fig. 4).

(b) **Keratosis obturans** (Fig. 5) is one of the closest differentials to EACC (Table 1).

(c) **Medial canal fibrosis** is another close differential for EACC. Patients usually have a significant history of chronic inflammatory ear disease and/or prior instrumentation or surgery. Otoscopically, the EAC is shallow, with the clinician often describing it as a pseudo-fundus. Radiologically, the lack of

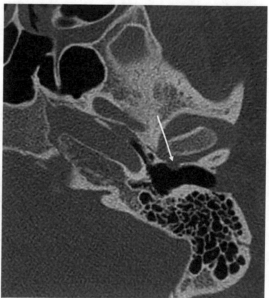

Fig. 3 Axial CT image shows the foramen of Huschke along the anterior wall of the EAC with a small amount of soft tissue (probably synovium or fat) herniating through this defect

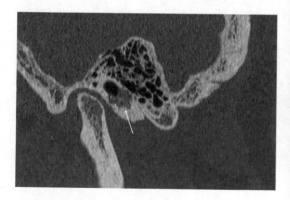

Fig. 2 Sagittal CT image of a patient with otalgia shows smooth erosions with intramural bone fragments involving the postero-inferior walls of the EAC (arrow) but without any significant intraluminal soft tissue component. Histology confirmed EAC cholesteatoma

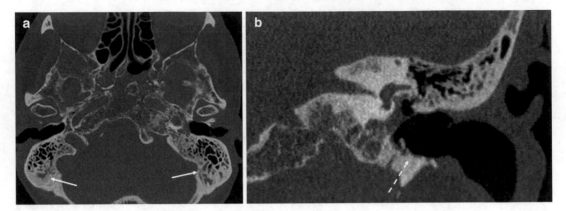

Fig. 4 (**a** and **b**) Axial (**a**) and coronal (**b**) CT images of a patient with prior history of nasopharyngeal carcinoma and radiotherapy, now presenting with left-sided otalgia. Axial image shows widespread skull base mottling, trabecular thickening and periosteal reaction along the mastoid air cell septae (arrows) compatible with radiotherapy-induced changes. Coronal image of the left EAC shows erosions along the floor of the EAC with a small bone fragment, note the absence of any significant soft tissue component. Features are consistent with osteoradionecrosis

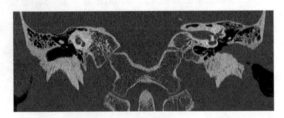

Fig. 5 Coronal CT image shows left-sided keratosis obturans. Note the smooth widening of the EAC (compared to contralateral normal side) with the distinct lack of any intramural bone fragments or adjacent wall erosions which differentiates it from EACC

Table 1 Differentiating features between EACC and keratosis obturans

EACC	Keratosis obturans
Otorrhea and dull otalgia	Acute severe otalgia and CHL
Unilateral	Bilateral (usually)
Normal calibre EAC	Occluded and widened EACs
Bony erosions	No erosions
Intramural bone fragments (present in ~50%)	Soft tissue plugs without internal bone fragments

any bony changes is the main differentiating feature (refer Sect. 2 in chapter 'Imaging of External Ear Malformations, Canal Stenosis and Exostosis').

> **What the Surgeon Wants to Know?**
>
> - Degree of EACC extension into the middle ear cavity
> - Any involvement of the mastoid air cells
> - Is the integrity of the facial nerve canal and tegmen mastoideum preserved?

2 External Auditory Canal Malignant Neoplasms

2.1 What Malignancy Affects the EAC?

Malignant neoplasm of the EAC is very rare; squamous cell carcinoma (SCC) is the most common malignancy of the EAC followed distantly by adenocarcinoma. Secondary EAC involvement from adjacent skin SCC is more common than primary SCC of the EAC itself.

2.2 Clinical Features and Management

Patients (fifth and sixth decades) present with an ulcerative external ear and EAC lesion, otorrhoea, otalgia and conductive hearing loss. There is a high association with previous head and neck radiotherapy.

EAC malignancy can mimic benign processes like EACC and MOE on imaging, as these too present with soft tissue lesions in the EAC with surrounding bony changes. Malignancy should be considered in any adult having an EAC lesion with bony destruction, especially in those without a history of diabetes mellitus. EAC carcinomas are treated with surgical resection (±radiation and chemotherapy). As such, local tumour extent at presentation is the single most important factor determining survival.

2.3 Choice of Imaging

EAC malignancy can mimic other conditions as detailed earlier, but the real purpose of imaging is rarely diagnosis but rather delineating the extent of confirmed disease.

Contrast-enhanced MRI is the imaging modality of choice for delineation of local tumour extent, spread along neurovascular pathways, assessment of the deep neck spaces and intracranial extension. High-resolution CT of the temporal bone is superior in demonstrating bony involvement (Fig. 6).

2.4 Imaging Appearances

SCC frequently involves both cartilaginous and bony parts of the EAC, whereas adenocarcinoma tends to spare the bony segment. EAC wall erosions and extension into the adjacent spaces are common and can be seen on CT imaging as well (Fig. 7). On MR, EAC malignancies follow stan-

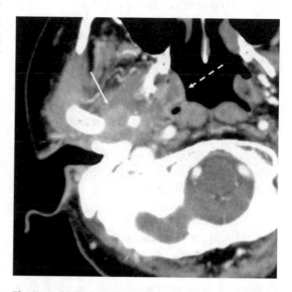

Fig. 7 Axial CT image of a patient with confirmed SCC of the EAC shows extension into the anterior masticator space (arrow) and medial nasopharyngeal space (dashed arrow)

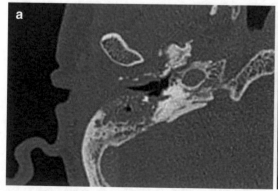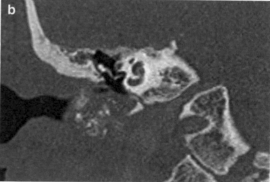

Fig. 6 (**a** and **b**) Axial and coronal CT images of a patient with verrucous SCC show gross bony destruction of the anterior and posterior walls of the EAC with extension into the underlying mastoid segment. Note the numerous bone fragments within the destructive soft tissue lesion, which could be easily mistaken for EACC in another clinical context (presence of squames on otoscopy)

dard imaging appearance of most head and neck malignancy, i.e. lobular, infiltrating mass that demonstrates restricted diffusion, intermediate to low T1WI and heterogeneous high T2WI intensity with enhancement (refer Sect. 2 in chapter 'Radiological Features of Otitis Externa'). Tumour necrosis is uncommon.

2.5 Differentials

The condition that mimics squamous cell carcinoma of the EAC most closely is MOE (refer Sect. 2 in chapter 'Radiological Features of Otitis Externa'), as both show similar bony changes and spread to the deep spaces of the neck. A history of diabetes mellitus and the presence of abscesses would favour MOE over squamous cell carcinoma of the EAC. The imaging appearances of other EAC carcinomas may also mimic MOE as well as EACC and ORN.

2.6 What the Surgeon Wants to Know?

Given that these lesions are easily sampled, diagnosis has usually been established prior to most imaging. The surgeon's primary concern remains assessment of the local disease extent and possible distal involvement.

Checklist for EAC Malignancy
- Extension across the tympanic membrane into the middle ear structures is rare (decreases the 5-year survival rate by ~50%)
- Superficial extension: Adjacent scalp, external ear/pinna, parotid gland
- Local extension: Degree of EAC involvement, i.e. superficial skin, cartilage or bony walls
- Anterior extension—TMJ
- Medial extension—Parapharyngeal spaces, middle ear, facial nerve canal
- Posterior extension—Mastoid

- Superior extension—Middle cranial fossa (intra-cranial)
- Inferior extension—Deep spaces of the neck
- Lymph node disease: Intraparotid nodes (first station), pre- and post-auricular nodes

3 Summary for External Auditory Canal Soft Tissue Lesions

Summary for EAC soft tissue lesions

Bone changes	Associated condition	Remember
Focal erosions	EAC cholesteatoma	Look for bone fragments within the soft tissue component
Diffuse canal widening	Keratosis obturans	Soft tissue occludes both canals almost completely
Destructive bony changes	MOE or EAC malignancy	Background diabetes and abscesses favour MOE
No bony changes	Medial canal fibrosis	'Pseudo-fundus'

Further Reading

Chawla A, Bosco JI, Lim TC, Shenoy JN, Krishnan V (2015) Computed tomography features of external auditory canal cholesteatoma: a pictorial review. Curr Probl Diagn Radiol 44(6):511–516

Heilbrun ME, Salzman KL, Glastonbury CM, Harnsberger HR, Kennedy RJ, Shelton C (2003) External auditory canal cholesteatoma: clinical and imaging spectrum. Am J Neuroradiol 24(4):751–756

Ong CK, Pua U, Chong VF (2008) Imaging of carcinoma of the external auditory canal: a pictorial essay. Cancer Imaging 8(1)

Xia S, Yan S, Zhang M, Cheng Y, Noel J, Chong V, Shen W (2015) Radiological findings of malignant tumours of external auditory canal: a cross-sectional study between squamous cell carcinoma and adenocarcinoma. Medicine 94(35)

Imaging of External Ear Malformations, Canal Stenosis and Exostosis

Tahira Kumar and Geoiphy George Pulickal

Contents

Abstract

This chapter summarizes congenital aural dysplasia, and a surgically relevant checklist is provided to aid in reporting. Subsequently, an overview of stenosing conditions that affect the external ear canal is given; i.e. medial canal fibrosis, exostoses and osteoma. Their differentiating features are enumerated, and pictorial examples are provided.

T. Kumar · G. G. Pulickal (✉)
Department of Diagnostic Radiology, Khoo Teck Puat Hospital, Singapore, Singapore
e-mail: kumar.tahira.sultana@ktph.com.sg; pulickal.george.geoiphy@ktph.com.sg

1 Congenital Aural Dysplasia (CAD)

1.1 Overview of Congenital Aural Dysplasia

Since the external and middle ear have a common embryological origin (first branchial apparatus), congenital anomalies tend to involve both.

CAD results due to failure of the first branchial cleft to canalize, causing varying degrees of stenosis (Fig. 1) to complete absence (atresia) of the external ear canal (EAC) (Fig. 2). In EAC atresia, this failure of tympanic bone canalization results in bone overgrowth and deformity, which is referred to as the "atresia (or atretic) plate".

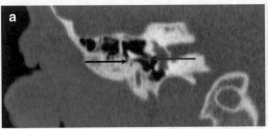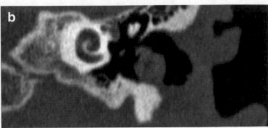

Fig. 1 (**a** and **b**) Coronal CT images of (**a**) right-sided bony atresia and (**b**) left-sided fibrotic stenosis of EAC in a 7-year-old boy. The malleus–incus complex is dysplastic with hammer handle attached to atretic bony plate on the right side (black arrow). Note the dehiscent facial nerve (red arrow) and auricle abnormality. There is bulky plug like soft tissue in the left EAC causing membranous stenosis in an otherwise unremarkable middle and inner ear

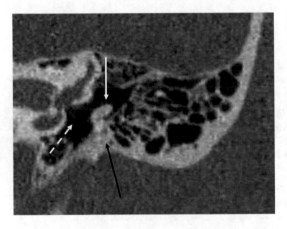

Fig. 2 Coronal CT scan shows complete atresia of the left EAC with a thick bony atretic plate (black arrow). The middle ear cavity appears well pneumatized, the deformed incudomalleolar complex (white arrow) is fused to the atretic plate and parts of the stapes superstructure (white dashed arrow) and oval window are visualized

Lesser branchiogenic anomalies can occur around the external ear in the form of cyst, sinus or fistula. Another common anomaly is a "pre-auricular sinus" (unrelated to the first branchial apparatus) that is diagnosed clinically. It is located around the anterior crus of the helix and is usually asymptomatic. It may get repeatedly infected and may lead to chronic discharge, abscess formation and scarring. The diagnosis is suspected clinically in presence of auricular deformities at birth or early childhood. Unilateral EAC stenosis without any auricular involvement may remain undiagnosed till adult life.

> **Tip**
> - *The "pre-auricular sinus" might be one of the rare instances in temporal bone imaging, where a focused ultrasound to delineate the tract, branches or any collections prior to resection is probably better than cross-sectional imaging.*

1.2   What the Surgeon Wants to Know

The sensorineural component of hearing tends to be intact, and the affected conductive component can be restored surgically in some patients. Reconstruction is not normally considered until a child is 7 years of age. As the condition is clinically apparent, imaging is usually reserved for preoperative planning. Refer to the below preoperative checklist for details (Table 1).

2   Medial Canal Fibrosis (MCF)

MCF is an acquired occlusion of the medial EAC by fibrous tissue, most commonly due to chronic otitis media or externa. Inflammatory granulation tissue progressively accumulates lateral to the tympanic membrane and eventually forms a fibrous plug.

Table 1 Congenital EAC atresia checklist

Auricle	Auricular deformities
Type	Bony, membranous, or mixed
Atretic plate	Complete or incomplete, measure thickness
Pneumatization	Pneumatization/opacification of middle ear and mastoid bone, width of middle ear cavity from atretic plate to promontory
Ear ossicles	Malleus-incus-stapes may be normal or dysplastic depending on degree of microtia
Cholesteatoma	Soft tissue in non-pneumatized portion with evidence of expansion and/or erosion
Facial nerve	Particularly, the course of tympanic and mastoid segment. Does the nerve pass across the tympanic cavity, along or through the atretic plate?
Oval and round windows	Open or occluded (contraindication for surgery)
Inner ear abnormality	Uncommon in isolated atresia
Anatomy of skull base	Low middle cranial fossa, anomalous course of ICA, large jugular bulb, TMJ in contact/proximity to the tympanic cavity etc.

2.1 Clinical Features and Management

Patients present with a chronically discharging ear and then with conductive hearing loss. Otoscopic examination reveals a blind-ending fundus (Fig. 3). The standard treatment is surgical resection of the occluding fibrous tissue down to the tympanic membrane and placement of split skin graft. Re-stenosis is of clinical concern.

2.2 Imaging Appearance

In the early stages, only mild thickening of the tympanic membrane is evident. Progressively thicker crescentic soft tissue will be seen filling in the EAC (Fig. 4). Important negative findings include a lack of bony erosions, canal wall expansion and intramural calcifications, which help differentiate this condition from EAC cholesteatoma (EACC) and keratosis obturans.

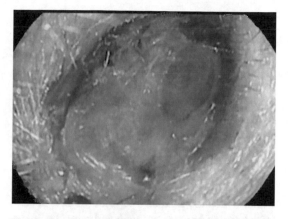

Fig. 3 Otoscopic image of a patient complaining of conductive hearing loss shows a "pseudo or false fundus" with soft tissue obliterating the medial end of the EAC prematurely and obscuring the normal tympanic membrane and handle of malleus. (Courtesy Dr. Amanda Cheang)

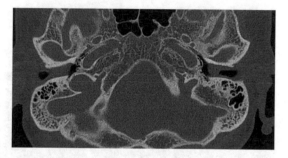

Fig. 4 Axial CT image shows bilateral EAC occlusion by concentric soft tissue, thicker on right. Note the absence of any concomitant bony erosions, intramural bone fragments or widening of the EAC

2.3 What the Surgeon Needs to Know

What the Surgeon Wants to Know

- Thickness and length of the fibrous plug/disc
- Composition of the fibrous plug, any bony component?
- Anything behind the false fundus?
- Any cholesteatoma?
- Presence of tympanosclerosis (e.g. post-inflammatory ossicular fixation) or congenital anomalies which could impact the hearing outcome
- Important anatomical variations like aberrant ICA or facial nerve course etc.

3   Exostoses

Exostoses refer to lamellar bone deposition along the external ear canal that narrows it. It is usually the result of chronic irritation, classically thermal—cold water exposure (hence referred to as surfer's or swimmer's ear).

3.1   Clinical Features and Management

Patients usually in their 30s and 40s can present with hearing impairment, pain and repetitive infection (when the self-cleaning mechanism of the EAC has been obstructed sufficiently). Otoscopy reveals a narrow external auditory canal with a barely visualized intact tympanic membrane.

Initial treatment is aimed at avoiding further exposure and treating the presenting symptoms;

if unsuccessful, then definite surgical treatment is transmeatal excision of the exostoses.

3.2   Imaging Appearance

On CT (which is the imaging of choice), exostoses appear as broad-based dense bony protuberances arising medial to the isthmus (focal narrowing of the EAC about 6 mm lateral to the tympanic membrane) causing stenosis of the canal (Fig. 5).

3.3   Exostoses Vs. Osteoma

The only other entity for which exostoses can realistically be mistaken for is osteoma (Table 2) (Fig. 6).

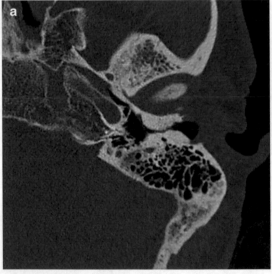
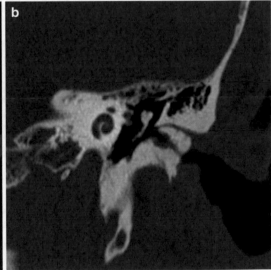

Fig. 5 (**a** and **b**) Axial (**a**) and coronal (**b**) CT images of a patient with bilateral hearing loss show a well-defined broad-based bony lesion in the medial aspect of the left EAC causing severe stenosis. Similar right-sided findings were noted as well (not shown). (Courtesy Dr. Thi Nguyen, Benson Radiology, Adelaide)

Table 2 Osseous EAC stenosis

Exostoses	Osteoma
Cold water exposure	Often incidental
Bilateral	Unilateral
Sessile broad based	Pedunculated and usually solitary
Medial to isthmus	Lateral to isthmus

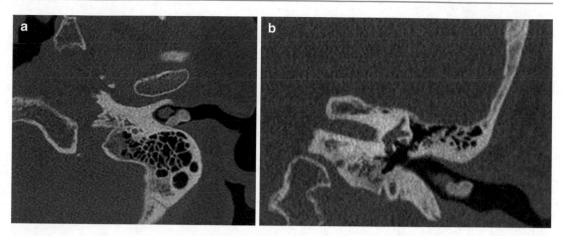

Fig. 6 (**a** and **b**) Axial (**a**) and coronal CT (**b**) images show a well-defined pedunculated osteoma in the lateral aspect of the left EAC with build-up of cerumen behind it

Further Reading

Baumgartner BJ, Backous DD (2006) Radiology quiz case 1. Postinflammatory fibrosis of the EAC (medial canal fibrosis). Arch Otolaryngol Head Neck Surg 132(6):690, 692

Gassner EM, Mallouhi A, Jaschke WR (2004) Preoperative evaluation of external auditory canal atresia on high-resolution CT. AJR Am J Roentgenol 182(5):1305–1312

Swartz JD, Faerber EN (1985) Congenital malformations of the external and middle ear: high-resolution CT findings of surgical import. AJR Am J Roentgenol 144(3):501–506

Turetsky DB, Vines FS, Clayman DA (1990) Surfer's ear: exostoses of the external auditory canal. AJNR Am J Neuroradiol 11(6):1217–1218

Part III

Imaging of Middle Ear and Mastoid Air Cells; Pathology

Imaging of Otomastoiditis: Acute and Chronic

Julian Sau Lian Chieng

Contents

Abstract

This chapter explains the clinical and imaging features of otomastoiditis, both acute and chronic forms. Special attention is given on how to discern and report on potential complications and causes of associated hearing loss. Quick reference pre-surgical checklist is provided as well.

J. S. L. Chieng (✉)
Department of Diagnostic Radiology, Woodlands
Healthcare Campus, Singapore, Singapore
e-mail: julian_chieng@whc.sg

1 Acute Otomastoiditis

Otomastoiditis is the inflammation of the middle ear (otitis media) and mastoid (mastoiditis). Acute otitis media is primarily a disease of infants and young children.

The middle ear, mastoid air cells and pneumatized petrous bone are extensions of the upper respiratory tract. Reflux of infected secretions from the nasopharynx through the Eustachian tube (often incompetent in children) permits the entry of bacteria into the middle ear cavity and beyond. *Streptococcus pneumoniae* and *Haemophilus influenza* are the most common causative bacteria.

© Springer Nature Switzerland AG 2021
G. G. Pulickal et al. (eds.), *Temporal Bone Imaging Made Easy*,
Medical Radiology Diagnostic Imaging, https://doi.org/10.1007/978-3-030-70635-7_12

1.1 Clinical Features and Management

Patients with uncomplicated acute otitis media present with fever, otalgia and red bulging tympanic membrane. Fluid accumulation in the middle ear cavity could progress from serous to purulent and the tympanic membrane may rupture, resulting in decompression of the middle ear cavity and otorrhea. If the patient has concurrent mastoiditis (which invariably is the case), then retro-auricular swelling, erythema and tenderness may be present.

The clinical course of uncomplicated acute otomastoiditis is usually short and is treated effectively with antibiotics. Surgical intervention (e.g. myringotomy with or without ventilation tube) is considered in selected cases, e.g. patients who have severe otalgia or appear toxic.

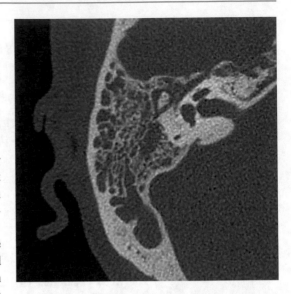

Fig. 1 Axial CT image of uncomplicated acute otomastoiditis shows opacification of middle ear cavity and mastoid air cells with preservation of the ossicular chain, trabeculae and mastoid cortical bones

1.2 Choice of Imaging and Imaging Features

Diagnosis is made clinically, and imaging is only indicated if bone disease is suspected.

The imaging technique of choice usually is high-resolution CT of the temporal bone.

Uncomplicated disease shows opacification of the middle ear, mastoid antrum and air cells without any bony erosion and preservation of the ossicular chain (Fig. 1).

With bone disease, periosteal reaction and erosions of the mastoid trabeculae and cortices are seen resulting in coalescent mastoiditis (Fig. 2). Intravenous contrast is only needed if associated peri-mastoid collections are suspected. MR imaging is usually reserved for detection or detailed evaluation of intracranial complications.

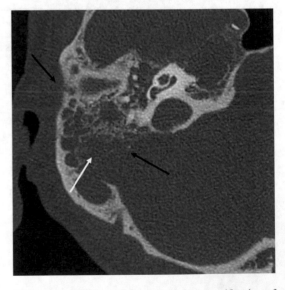

Fig. 2 Axial CT image shows complete opacification of the middle ear cavity and mastoid air cells. Erosions of the trabecular septae (white arrow) and cortical bone of the mastoid (black arrows) are compatible with coalescent mastoiditis

1.3 Complications

Small proportion of untreated or inadequately treated patients may experience complications (Table 1). Intra-temporal/extra-cranial complications predominate over intracranial complications.

Intra-temporal/extracranial complications

1. **Coalescent mastoiditis**
   CT demonstrates erosion of the honeycomb-like trabecular septa of the

mastoid and/or erosion of the mastoid cortical bone (Fig. 2).

2. **Subperiosteal abscess**

   When pus within the mastoid bursts through the external cortex and lies underneath the periosteum, a subperiosteal abscess is formed. It may be postauricular, extend towards the external auditory canal or along the zygomatic bone.

3. **Bezold abscess**

   When the infection spreads into the substance of the sternocleidomastoid/digastric muscles (via their attachment sites at the mastoid tip) and forms an abscess, it is referred to as a "Bezold abscess" (Fig. 3).

4. **Petrous apicitis**

   The infection may extend anteriorly to involve the pneumatized petrous apex, which shows opacification and sometimes erosion. Gradenigo syndrome is the classical presentation of petrous apicitis (triad of otorrhea, sixth nerve palsy and deep facial pain) (refer Sect.

5 in chapter "Imaging of the Petrous Apex, Cerebellopontine Angles and Jugular Foramen").

5. **Facial nerve palsy**

   This is a rare but often reversible complication, commonly affecting the tympanic and upper mastoid segments of the facial nerve. Erosion along the facial nerve canal may not always be readily visible, and palsy can occur without any obvious involvement of the facial nerve canal. On MR imagining, abnormal enhancement along the nerve may be visible (refer Sect. 5 in chapter "Imaging of the Facial Nerve: Approach and Pathology").

6. **Labyrinthitis**

   Infection can spread into the labyrinth via preformed pathways, such as round or oval windows or by direct invasion of the bony labyrinth, resulting in suppurative labyrinthitis (refer Sect. 4 in chapter "Other Causes of Inner Ear Hearing Loss: Meniere's Disease, Labyrinthitis and Semicircular Canal Dehiscence").

Table 1 Local and intracranial complications

Intratemporal complications	Intracranial complications
Coalescent mastoiditis	Intracranial abscess (epidural, subdural, intracerebral)
Subperiosteal and Bezold abscess	Dural venous thrombophlebitis (sigmoid and transverse)
Petrous apicitis	Meningitis/encephalitis
Labyrinthitis	
Facial nerve paralysis	

2 Chronic Otomastoiditis

Chronic otomastoiditis (COM) is persistent inflammation of the middle ear cavity and mastoid for at least 12 weeks. The primary aetiology is that of Eustachian tube dysfunction, resulting in a chronic negative intra-tympanic pressure. This gives rise to various manifestations, such as tympanic membrane

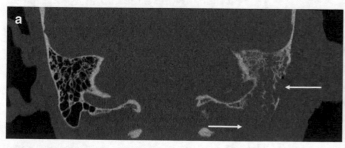
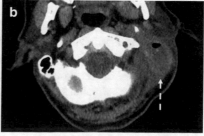

Fig. 3 (**a** and **b**) Bone window coronal (**a**) and soft tissue window axial (**b**) CT images of a patient with severe mastoiditis show almost complete erosion of the mastoid tip and cortex (arrows) and gas-forming loculated collection immediately beneath it, involving the sternocleidomastoid muscle (dashed arrow). Note the normal contralateral side for comparison

perforation/retraction, effusion, granulation tissue, cholesterol granuloma, cholesteatoma, ossicular fixation and post-inflammatory ossicular erosions (ossicular erosions without cholesteatoma).

2.1 Clinical Features and Management

Patients present with otorrhea and hearing impairment (usually conductive hearing loss). On otoscopic examination, a perforated and/or retracted tympanic membrane is seen along with various combination of fluid, granulation tissue, mucosal polyps, ossicular erosions, ossicular fixation (post-inflammatory ossicular fixation), cholesterol granuloma or cholesteatoma within the middle ear.

The primary treatment modality is a combination of aural toilet and topical antimicrobial drops. Surgical approaches include mastoidectomy and tympanoplasty. If the patient develops cholesteatoma, surgical eradication of the cholesteatoma is indicated.

2.2 Choice of Imaging

Imaging in COM is indicated if the long-standing inflammation is unresponsive to medical treatment for evaluation of hearing loss (ossicular erosion or fixation), clinical suspicion of cholesteatoma or suspected intratemporal or intracranial complications, similar to acute otomastoiditis.

CT of the temporal bone is the imaging of choice to evaluate the ossicular chain, walls of the middle ear cavity and mastoid. MRI can play a role in the detection of (primary or residual) cholesteatoma, cholesterol granuloma or when intracranial complications are suspected.

2.3 Imaging Features

A chronically inflamed middle ear cleft will result in obstruction and loss of normal aera-

tion which in turn can give rise to osteitis, new bone formation and hyalinization/calcification, which are the imaging hallmarks of COM. These changes can be seen along the tympanic membrane in the middle ear cavity and mastoid.

2.3.1 Tympanic Membrane

The normal tympanic membrane (TM) is barely perceptible on CT imaging. Any process that causes the TM to be thicker, i.e. more conspicuous, is abnormal (Fig. 4). The TM can be perforated and/or retracted, both being better appreciated on otoscopy. Hyalinization and calcification along the TM are referred to as myringosclerosis.

2.3.2 Middle Ear Cavity

Granulation tissue can be seen in COM appearing as a non-dependent soft tissue opacification in the middle ear cavity, usually without ossicular displacement or bone erosion (Fig. 5). It can be indistinguishable from effusion or cholesteoma on CT but often occurs concurrently with these.

An effusion can only be diagnosed on CT imaging if an air-fluid level is seen. In the presence of complete opacification of the middle ear, mastoid antrum and air cells (the holotympanic opacity), it would not be possible to differentiate between fluid from solid substances like granulation tissue, as such it is important to report the presence of an effusion only if air–fluid levels are clearly seen. If the opacification is due to granulation tissue but mis-reported as an effusion, this might lead to the unnecessary placement of a grommet tube by the clinician. In holotympanic opacity, it is better to state that there is uncertainty whether the opacity is due to fluid or granulation tissue or a combination of both, rather than calling it as an effusion. *(Changes along the ossicular chain will be discussed separately later in the chapter)*

2.3.3 Mastoid Temporal Bone

The affected mastoid portion of the temporal bone shows sclerosis with under pneumatization of the mastoid air cells, frequently with opacification of the remnant air cells (Fig. 5).

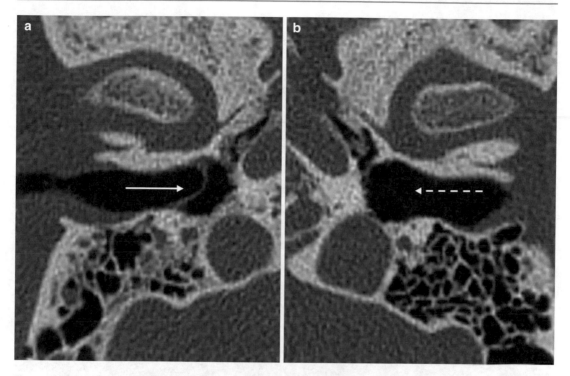

Fig. 4 (**a** and **b**) Axial CT images show a clearly visibly thickened right tympanic membrane (arrow), note the contralateral normal side where the tympanic membrane is barely visible (dashed arrow)

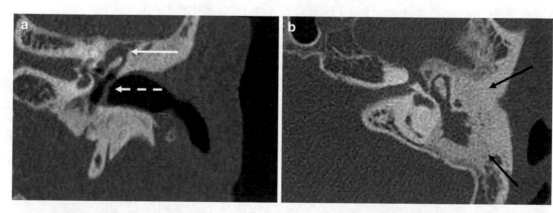

Fig. 5 (**a** and **b**) Coronal (**a**) and axial (**b**) CT images of a patient with COM show non-dependent opacification of the epitympanum and mastoid antrum (white arrow). Note the additional myringosclerosis (dashed arrow), back-ground sclerosis and profound under pneumatization of the mastoid air cells (black arrows) are suggestive of long-standing inflammation

2.4 Hearing Loss in Chronic Otomastoiditis

Hearing loss in CMO is usually conductive in nature with either fixation or erosion of the ossicular chain, leading to interrupted sound transmission.

2.4.1 Post-inflammatory Ossicular Chain Fixation

Post-inflammatory ossicular chain fixation (PIOF) is divided into three pathologic forms: fibrous tissue fixation, tympanosclerosis and fibro-osseous sclerosis (Table 2) (Figs. 6, 7 and 8). The imaging features of fibrous fixation are

Table 2 Types of post-inflammatory ossicular chain fixation

Type	Feature	Common location	Remember
Fibrous tissue fixation	Non-calcified soft tissue densities around some/all of the ossicular chain	Oval window involvement resulting in stapes fixation	Involvement of the Prussak's space can mimic cholesteatoma
Tympanosclerosis	Focal calcifications along the TM, tendons, ossicular surface (thickening) or ossicular ligaments	TM is commonly involved → Myringosclerosis	Myringosclerosis can be asymptomatic
Fibro-osseous sclerosis	New lamellar bone structures of high density causing thick bony webs or generalized encasement	Propensity for the epitympanum	Least common sub-type of PIOF

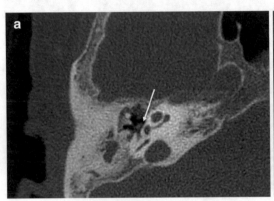

Fig. 6 (**a** and **b**) Axial (**a**) and coronal (**b**) CT images of a patient with conductive hearing loss show soft tissue opacification around the stapes and oval window (arrows). Note the non-dependent opacification in the epitympa-

num, background mastoid sclerosis and under pneumatization. Findings are compatible with fibrous tissue fixation of the stapes secondary to chronic otomastoiditis

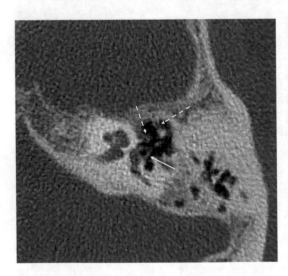

Fig. 7 Axial CT image of a patient with chronic otomastoiditis shows increased sclerosis along the stapes (arrow) as well as calcifications along the tensor tympani tendon and the anterior malleus ligament (dashed arrows). Findings are compatible with tympanosclerosis

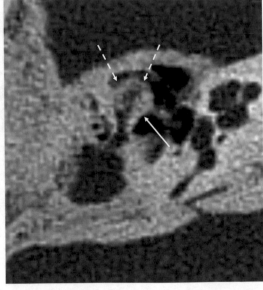

Fig. 8 Axial CT image shows Fibro-osseous sclerosis with thick lamellar bone formation (dashed arrows) in the epitympanum partially encasing the incudomalleolar complex (arrow)

non-specific, usually showing the presence of non-calcified soft tissue around some or all of the intact ossicles. The diagnosis of fibrous fixation is only made if there is a corresponding wide air-bone gap of more than 30 decibels on audiometry.

Post-inflammatory ossicular chain erosion is less common than erosion caused by cholesteatoma. If erosive changes do occur, these are in order of decreasing frequency: along the long process incus, crura of stapes, body of the incus and manubrium of malleus.

2.4.2 Cholesteatoma and Chronic Otomastoiditis

Acquired cholesteatoma is seen in the setting of COM and often coexists with granulation tissue. There are some clinical and radiological features that favour cholesteatoma over granulation tissue (Table 3). However, it must be pointed out that the diagnosis of cholesteatoma is made more often clinically than radiologically by the presence of squames or a pearly white mass (refer Sect. 3 in chapter "Radiological Features of Acquired and Congenital Cholesteatoma").

2.5 What the Surgeon Wants to Know

Surgical treatment is aimed at clearing the disease, preventing any potential complications and, if possible, restoring or at least improving hear-

ing. Surgical interventions can extend from simple tympanoplasties to complex ossicular chain reconstructions with varying types of mastoidectomies. In pre-surgical imaging, the following points need to be highlighted.

Checklist for Otitis Media
- Has there been any prior surgery or is the mastoid anatomy significantly altered?
- What is the degree of mastoid pneumatization, opacification or sclerosis?
- Any suggestion of PIOF?
- Is the ossicular chain eroded?
- Is there a cholesteatoma? If yes, are there any complications? (e.g. erosion of the tegmen tympani/mastoideum, facial nerve canal and bony labyrinth-labyrinthine fistula)?
- Are there any normal variants that may pose a surgical risk? (e.g. low tegmen tympani, laterally displaced sigmoid sinus, facial nerve canal dehiscence, high-riding and dehiscent jugular bulb with part of the internal jugular vein protruding into the middle ear cavity)

Table 3 Granulation tissues vs. cholesteatoma

Features	Granulation tissue	Cholesteatoma
Otoscopy	Inflamed tissue that often bleeds on contact, may be polypoidal	Presence of squames
Middle ear cleft opacification and sclerosis	Often	Often
Bony erosions	Infrequent	Frequent
Mass effect	Usually none	Common

Further Reading

Hoeffner EG (2008) Chronic otitis media. In: Hoeffner EG, Mukherji SK (eds) Temporal bone imaging. Thieme, New York, pp 67–70

Mittal R, Lisi CV, Gerring R, Mittal J, Mathee K, Narasimhan G, Azad RK, Yao Q, Grati MH, Yan D, Eshraghi AA (2015) Current concepts in the pathogenesis and treatment of chronic suppurative otitis media. J Med Microbiol 64(10):1103–1116

Nemzek WR, Swartz JD (2003) Temporal bone: inflammatory disease. In: Som PM, Curtin HD (eds) Head and neck imaging, 4th edn. Mosby, St Louis, pp 1173–1229

Saat R, Laulajainen-Hongisto AH, Mahmood G, Lempinen LJ, Aarnisalo AA, Jero J et al (2015) MR imaging features of acute mastoiditis and their clinical relevance. AJNR Am J Neuroradiol 36:361–367

Trojanowska A, Drop A, Trojanowski P, Rosińska-Bogusiewicz K, Klatka J, Bobek-Billewicz B (2012) External and middle ear diseases: radiological diagnosis based on clinical signs and symptoms. Insights Imaging 3(1):33–48

Vazquez E, Castellote A, Piqueras J, Mauleon S, Creixell S, Pumarola F, Figueras C, Carreño JC (2003) Lucaya J. Imaging of complications of acute mastoiditis in children. Radiographics 23(2):359–372

Radiological Features of Acquired and Congenital Cholesteatoma

Alvin Yong Quan Soon
and Geoiphy George Pulickal

Contents

Abstract

This chapter provides a detailed summary of middle ear cholesteatoma. Clinical and imaging differences between acquired and congenital forms are highlighted, and potential differential diagnoses are explored. Quick summary of surgically relevant reporting points is provided as well.

A. Y. Q. Soon
Department of Diagnostic Radiology, Tan Tock Seng Hospital, Singapore, Singapore
e-mail: alvin_yq_soon@ttsh.com.sg

G. G. Pulickal (✉)
Department of Diagnostic Radiology, Khoo Teck Puat Hospital, Singapore, Singapore
e-mail: pulickal.george.geoiphy@ktph.com.sg

1   What Is a Cholesteatoma

A cholesteatoma is a benign inflammatory mass in the temporal bone comprising of an external layer stratified squamous epithelium (essentially skin) that continues to shed keratin debris into the middle of the lesion causing it to 'grow' continually. This results in periostitis and erosions along

© Springer Nature Switzerland AG 2021
G. G. Pulickal et al. (eds.), *Temporal Bone Imaging Made Easy*,
Medical Radiology Diagnostic Imaging, https://doi.org/10.1007/978-3-030-70635-7_13

the adjacent bone. Despite its invasive nature, it is not a tumour and does not contain any 'cholesterol' as its name erroneously suggests; in fact, histologically it is similar to epidermoid cysts seen in the posterior fossa.

2   Classification

Cholesteatomas can be classified according to location – EAC, middle ear or petrous apex or as per origin (pathogenesis), i.e. congenital or acquired or location.

Acquired cholesteatoma occurs in the setting of chronic otomastoiditis (COM) secondary to Eustachian tube dysfunction. The resultant negative pressure in the tympanic cavity gives rise to 'retraction pockets' along the TM into the middle ear cavity which eventually fill-in and enlarge. Depending on the site of the retraction along the tympanic membrane, it can either be further sub-classified as 'pars flaccida' (more common) or 'pars tensa' cholesteatoma (Fig. 1).

Congenital cholesteatoma can be located anywhere in the temporal bone, from the EAC to the petrous apex, but most frequently in the middle ear.

Tip
- *Mural cholesteatoma are rare variants of acquired cholesteatoma. They are large lesions in the middle ear/mastoid eroding through to the bony EAC. As the content of the lesion discharges into the EAC only a 'rind or shell' is left along the margins of the cavity which appears similar to a post-surgical mastoidectomy cavity, this process is referred to as auto-mastoidectomy (Fig. 2).*

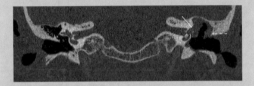

Fig. 2 Coronal CT image shows large left-sided cholesteatoma which has eroded through the bony EAC (dashed arrow) and discharged the bulk of the lesion (auto-mastoidectomy). A thick rind of soft tissue remains in the middle ear, note invasive nature of the cholesteatoma with involvement of the vestibule (arrow). Normal contralateral side for comparison

3   Clinical Features and Management

Congenital and acquired cholesteatomata present differently. Congenital cholesteatomata is usually seen in a younger age group and can be relatively asymptomatic. Presentation depends on its location, if situated in the middle ear cavity then with conductive hearing loss and if in the otic capsule then sensorineural hearing loss. On otoscopic evaluation, the classical description is that of a 'pearly white mass' behind an intact tympanic membrane.

Acquired cholesteatoma only occurs in the setting of chronic otomastoiditis (refer Sect. 3 in chapter 'Imaging of Otomastoiditis, Acute and Chronic'), as such the presentation is similar to COM. On otoscopy' a perforated tympanic membrane is usually encountered, with the presence of either a pearly white mass or squames (flakey

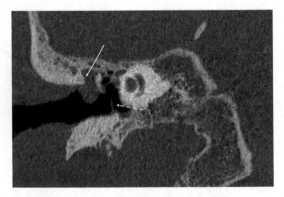

Fig. 1 Coronal CT image shows classical appearance of a pars flaccida cholesteatoma centered upon the Prussak's space. The soft tissue mass exerts considerable local mass effect displacing the malleus medially and eroding the scutum (arrow). Not the background changes of COM with sclerosis of the mastoid and a thickened and retracted tympanic membrane (dashed arrow)

white tissues) being diagnostic (refer Sect. 1 in chapter 'Common Otoscopic Signs, Imaging of Common Surgeries and Implants').

The management of cholesteatoma, whether congenital or acquired, consists of surgical resection and if possible restoration of the ossicular chain/hearing. Surgical clearance can be achieved by various types of mastoidectomies, each with their own advantages (refer Sect. 1 in chapter 'Common Otoscopic Signs, Imaging of Common Surgeries and Implants'). Surgical treatment could be done in stages with a 'second look' surgery traditionally being performed about a year after the initial surgical clearance to look for recurrence (though the rising availability of DWI MRI imaging is changing this practice).

4 Choice of Imaging

The diagnosis of cholesteatoma is usually made clinically. CT temporal bone is the initial imaging of choice to assess for its extent (although CT scan cannot differentiate cholesteatoma from adjacent granulation tissues), to evaluate the status of the ossicles (stapes being the most important), to rule out any complications (e.g. erosion of facial nerve canal, tegmen tympani/mastoideum, erosion of sinus plate and the presence of labyrinthine fistula) and look for any anatomical variants that can potentially be surgical hazards.

MRI is more specific in diagnosing cholesteatoma compared to CT. It is especially useful in the post-operative setting looking for recurrence and in clinically equivocal cases.

5 Imaging Features

The hallmarks of acquired cholesteatoma are that of a focal soft tissue opacity in a typical location (epitympanum and mastoid antrum), exerting local mass effect and causing adjacent bony ero-

sions. If this triad is present, then the likelihood of that soft tissue being cholesteatoma is extremely high, although it is important to note that not all cholesteatomata will show these constellations of findings. The temporal bone is usually sclerosed and under-pneumatized, with opacification of the mastoid air cells by fluid, granulation tissues or a combination of both (Fig. 1).

Pars flaccida subtypes are more common. The lesion will classically originate in the Prussak's space that lies immediately behind the pars flaccida (in the lateral epitympanic recess) (Fig. 1). The rarer pars tensa subtype lesion originates in the inferior aspect of the mesotympanum and will enlarge medially displacing the ossicular chain laterally. However, when the cholesteatoma is large, it is not possible to identify its point of origin.

Bony erosions are far less common in congenital lesions compared to acquired ones. Erosions usually involve the following structures: ossicles, scutum (for pars flaccida type and seen as a blunting), the walls of the middle ear cavity and mastoid antrum and, with advanced disease, the semi-circular canals, facial nerve canal and tegmen tympani may be involved as well (Figs. 2, 3 and 4).

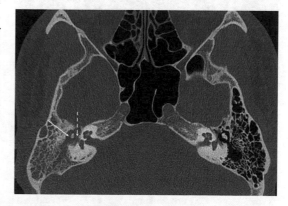

Fig. 3 Axial CT image of a patient with right-sided cholesteatoma shows opacification and widening of the epitympanum with typical erosions of the head of the malleus, body of the incus (arrow) and facial nerve canal (dashed arrow). The left side is normal

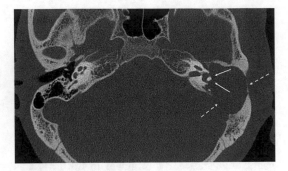

Fig. 4 Axial CT image shows a large left middle ear cholesteatoma that has eroded into the inner ear with involvement of the posterior semi-circular canal (arrows), the sigmoid plate and lateral cortex of the mastoid (dashed arrows). The ossicles have been completely eroded with no remnants being discerned with the mass

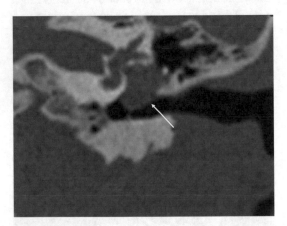

Fig. 5 Coronal CT image of young patient with hearing impairment shows a well-defined soft tissue mass in the middle ear cavity behind a normal intact tympanic membrane (arrow). Also note the well-aerated epitympanum/mastoid and well-defined scutum. Findings are compatible with a congenital cholesteatoma

The most common portion of the ossicular chain to be eroded is the long process of the incus, although this is non-specific, as it is also the most common site of erosion in non-cholesteatomatous lesions. Erosion of the malleus, the body of the incus and stapes are more common in cholesteatoma than in non-cholesteatomata ossicular erosion.

In congenital cholesteatoma, the classical 'white mass' seen on otoscopy usually corresponds to well-defined soft tissue opacity behind an intact TM (Fig. 5). The temporal bone is usually well-aerated, and if the lesion is in the middle ear, it is usually more inferiorly located than the acquired type, i.e. in the meso or hypotympanum instead of the epitympanum. Larger and advanced lesions will have similar clinical presentation and imaging features to acquired cholesteatoma. (Beyond the middle ear, congenital cholesteatoma may involve the geniculate ganglion (inner ear) or petrous apex (refer Sect. 5 in chapter 'Imaging of the Petrous Apex, Cerebellopontine Angles and Jugular Foramen') the major imaging differences between acquired and congenital cholesteatoma are enumerated below (Table 1).

> **Tip**
> • *The three hallmarks of cholesteatoma are typical location, mass effect and bone erosion.*

Table 1 Congenital vs acquired cholesteatoma

Type	Presentation	Tympanic membrane	Bony erosions	Location
Congenital cholesteatoma	Young patient presenting with hearing loss	Intac; white mass behind TM	Rare	Medial to ossicles
Acquired cholesteatoma	History of chronic ear discharge	Perforated and/or thickened; pearly white mass or squames in the EAC/Middle ear	Common	Pars flaccida → originates in Prussak's space Pars tensa → originates in inferior mesotympanum

MRI in Cholesteatoma: A Few Tips

- MRI protocols for cholesteatoma imaging vary across regions depending on the available technology and preference of the radiologist
- The restricted diffusion of the cholesteatoma keratin is the key finding in MRI imaging— *high SI on DWI and low on ADC* (Fig. 6)
- Possible mimics such as effusion, granulation tissue and inflammatory exudate return *high SI on ADC maps*
- Non-echoplanar imaging techniques have lesser air-bone artefacts than echoplanar acquisitions
- Coronal DWI and ADC maps are recommended
- Possible pitfalls include low keratin containing cholesteatoma (like mural cholesteatoma), small lesions (3 mm or less), proteinaceous fluid, post-operative material etc.
- Additional coronal T1- and T2-weighted images complimenting the DWI/ADC sequences are needed to overcome these pitfalls

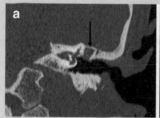 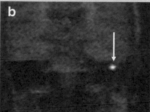 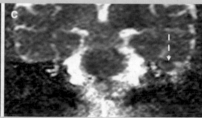

Fig. 6 (a–c) Coronal CT (**a**), MR DWI (**b**) and ADC (**c**) images of a known cholesteatoma patient with soft tissue in the post-operative mastoid cavity. On conventional CT image it is impossible to confidently specify this opacification (black arrow) as recurrent cholesteatoma, granulation tissue or retained secretions. MRI DWI image shows this lesion to have high signal intensity (white arrow) with corresponding hypointensity on the ADC image (dashed arrow), indicating restricted diffusion compatible with recurrent cholesteatoma. (Courtesy, Dr. Ravi Lingam, Northwick Park Hospital, London)

6   Differential Diagnosis

Important differentials for cholesteatoma in the middle ear are cholesterol granuloma, paraganglioma, facial nerve Schwannoma and aberrant ICA.

Cholesterol granuloma is far less common than cholesteatoma in the middle ear. Patients present with conductive hearing loss, and a bluish discoloration of the tympanic membrane is observed on otoscopy. CT shows a non-specific soft tissue opacity that cannot be differentiated from granulation tissues, usually without surrounding bony erosions. MRI is diagnostic, as the lesion shows characteristic T1 and T2 hyperintensity with facilitated diffusion, differentiating it clearly from possible cholesteatoma (T1 iso or hypointense with restricted diffusion).

Paraganglioma of the middle ear (glomus tympanicum) is a benign but locally invasive tumour. It is classically seen in middle-aged females who present with a history of pulsatile tinnitus or hearing loss. A pulsatile red (vascular) mass is seen behind an intact tympanic membrane. On CT imaging, it typically appears as a well-defined soft tissue mass overlying the cochlear promontory; associated bony erosions can be present but are not a consistent feature. MRI shows avid enhancement and larger lesions the distinctive 'salt and pepper' appearance (salt being the intra-lesional

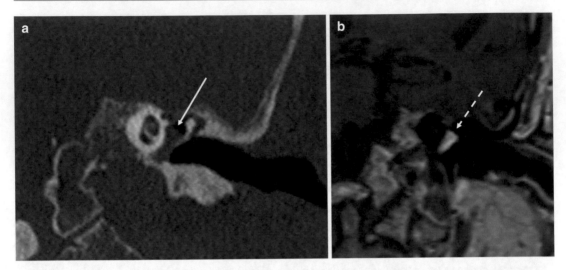

Fig. 7 (**a** and **b**) Coronal CT (**a**) and corresponding contrast-enhanced MR image (**b**) of a patient with left-sided pulsatile tinnitus shows well-defined soft tissue lesion over the cochlear promontory (arrow). On post-contrast MR imaging the lesion shows intense enhancement (dashed arrow). Findings are compatible with Glomus tympanicum

haemorrhage and the abundant vascular flow voids depicting pepper), like paragangliomas elsewhere (glomus jugulare, carotid body tumour etc.) (Fig. 7).

Middle ear Schwannomas typically arise from the tympanic segment of the facial nerve. Important imaging feature is that the mass is along the course of the facial nerve, and this helps to differentiate from cholesteatoma. Post-contrast MRI also depicts a strongly enhancing mass as opposed to cholesteatoma which does not enhance.

Aberrant ICA or high-riding jugular bulbs are readily diagnosed on CT or contrast-enhanced imaging and usually do not pose a diagnostic challenge on imaging.

What the Surgeon Wants to Know
- Describe the extent of the disease to facilitate complete clearance – the sinus tympani is a surgical blind spot
- Detail the ossicular chain disruption accurately to facilitate potential reconstructive surgery – most importantly the status of the stapes
- Tegmen tympani/mastoideum dehiscence/erosions – may lead to complication of meningitis and brain abscess, also there is increased risk of damaging the dura with potential CSF leak during and post surgery
- Facial nerve canal erosion – can lead to facial nerve palsy
- Labyrinthine fistula (erosion/involvement of the lateral semicircular canal, cochlear promontory, oval or round windows) – may cause Tullio phenomenon
- Sigmoid sinus plate involvement – may cause venous sinus thrombosis
- Important anatomical variations like low tegmen, anteriorly/laterally displaced sigmoid sinus, high and dehiscent jugular bulb, especially with protrusion into the middle ear.

Further Reading

Barath K, Huber AM, Stampfli P, Varga Z, Kollias S (2011) Neuroradiology of cholesteatomas. AJNR Am J Neuroradiol 32(2):221–229

Lingam RK, Nash R, Majithia A, Kalan A, Singh A (2016) Non-echoplanar diffusion weighted imaging in the detection of post-operative middle ear cholesteatoma: navigating beyond the pitfalls to find the pearl. Insights Imaging 7(5):669–678. https://doi.org/10.1007/s13244-016-0516-3. Epub 2016 Aug 24. Review

Koch BL, Hamilton BE, Hudgins PA, Harnsberger HR (2017) Diagnostic imaging head and neck, 3rd edn. Elsevier, Philadelphia

Radiological Features of Oval Window Atresia

Hau Wei Khoo and Tiong Yong Tan

Contents

Abstract

This chapter explains the clinical and radiological features of oval window atresia. Surgically relevant checklists and corresponding pictorial examples are provided for easy reference. Potential imaging mimics are discussed as well.

H. W. Khoo
Department of Diagnostic Radiology, Tan Tock Seng Hospital, Singapore, Singapore
e-mail: hauwei_khoo@ttsh.com.sg

T. Y. Tan (✉)
Department of Radiology, Changi General Hospital, Singapore, Singapore
e-mail: tan.tiong.yong@singhealth.com.sg

1 What Is Oval Window Atresia (or Absent Oval Window)?

It is a rare congenital cause of hearing loss due to the oval window failing to develop normally. It can occur by itself, but reported associations include Turner's and CHARGE syndromes.

2 Clinical Features and Management

Patients (typically children but some adults can present late) complain of hearing loss which is usually conductive or mixed type. Symptoms may be unilateral or bilateral, and there is no prior history of suppurative ear disease or progression of the hearing loss. External ear abnormalities may or may not be present as this condition can occur in isolation. Audiometry shows a large air-bone gap.

© Springer Nature Switzerland AG 2021
G. G. Pulickal et al. (eds.), *Temporal Bone Imaging Made Easy*,
Medical Radiology Diagnostic Imaging, https://doi.org/10.1007/978-3-030-70635-7_14

Treatment options include bone conduction hearing aid rehabilitation and surgical correction with vestibulotomy and prosthesis placement, with variable results.

3   Choice of Imaging

High-resolution CT of the temporal bone is the imaging of choice. MR imaging may be complementary in cases with sensorineural hearing loss to evaluate potential inner ear abnormalities (e.g., dysplasia of membranous labyrinth or vestibulocochlear nerve dysplasia).

4   Imaging Features

The oval window acts as the connection between the middle and the inner ear. It appears as a rectangular opening along the medial wall of the tympanic cavity and is best seen on the coronal plane, where its relation to the stapes is better appreciated (Fig. 1).

In oval window atresia, there is complete filling of the oval window by a thick bony plate or concentric narrowing with loss of the normal rectangular shape and only a dimple or wedge-like depression remaining along the medial tympanic wall (Fig. 2).

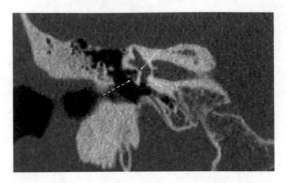

Fig. 2 Coronal CT image of a patient with profound right-sided hearing loss since birth secondary to atresia of the oval window. Note the loss of the normal rectangular configuration (wedge-shaped) and a thick bony plate covering the oval window (arrow). Note the aberrant course of the facial nerve lying over the promontory (dashed arrow)

The oval window is embryologically linked to the stapes footplate, annular ligament and the tympanic segment of the facial nerve. Thus, absent stapes footplate and an aberrant position of the tympanic segment of the facial nerve (typically inferiorly displacement to the level of the expected location of the oval window or cochlear promontory) being almost always present. Other dysplasia along the ossicular chain including the rest of the stapes superstructure and incus can coexist as well.

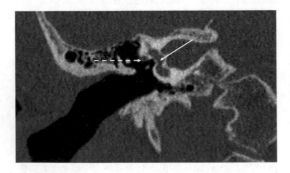

Fig. 1 Coronal CT image shows a normal rectangular shaped oval window (arrow) with the tympanic segment of the facial nerve lying superolateral to the oval window

What the Surgeon Wants to Know
- Any stapes superstructure and/or incus malformation that may affect prosthesis placement? (Fig. 3)
- Is the aberrant positioned facial nerve obstructing surgical access (if it overlies the expected location of the oval window)? (Fig. 4)
- Comment on patency of round window.
- Any associated external or inner ear malformations? (Fig. 5)

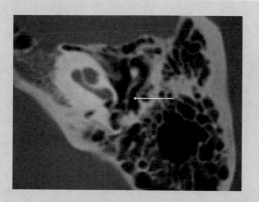

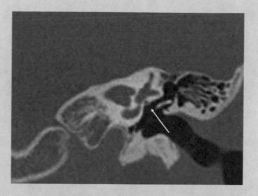

Fig. 3 Axial CT image of a patient with known oval window atresia shows stapes dysplasia (lack of a footplate) and inferior displacement of the incudostapedial articulation (arrow) due to the unopposed action of the stapedius muscle

Fig. 4 Coronal CT image of a patient with known oval window atresia shows inferior displacement of the tympanic segment of the facial nerve over the expected location of the oval window (arrow), precluding vestibulotomy

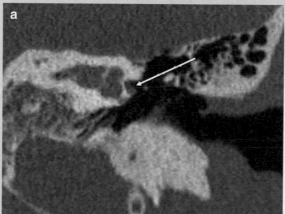

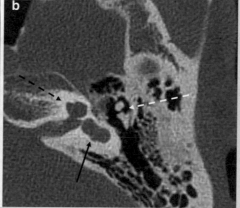

Fig. 5 Coronal (**a**) and axial (**b**) CT images of a patient with known oval window atresia showing characteristic inferior displacement of the facial nerve (white arrow). Along with the oval window atresia, significant inner ear malformations involving the cochlea, i.e., note the absent modiolus and lack of defined turns (dashed black arrow) and the semicircular canals (black arrow). Also note the deformed incus and malleoincudal dislocation (dashed white arrow)

5 Differentials

Fenestral otosclerosis could mimic oval window atresia with heaped up ground-glass density bone obliterating the oval window opening (Fig. 6).

Lack of ossicular chain dysplasia and normal course of the facial nerve are important differentiating features (refer Sect. 4 in chapter "Radiological Features of Otosclerosis").

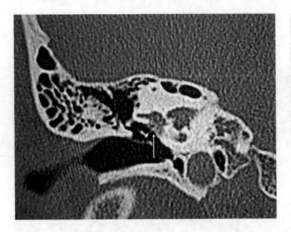

Fig. 6 Coronal CT image of a patient with conductive hearing loss shows a large hypodense otospongiotic plaque extending from the fissula ante fenestram to completely obliterate the oval window and fix the stapes (arrow). Note the typical ground-glass density of otospongiotic plaque

> **Tip**
> - *Stapes footplate fixation occurs due to the failure of formation of the annular ligament and is one of the commonest causes of congenital conductive hearing loss. Unfortunately, it is usually only diagnosed on exploratory tympanotomy, as the CT scan tends to be normal.*

Congenital ossicular chain fixation by bony bars, ossified/calcified ligaments or tendon, stapes footplate fixation, or severely protruded tympanic portion of the facial nerve.

Tympanosclerosis may be considered another differential, but a typical history of chronic ear discharge and corresponding inflammatory changes in the middle ear cleft should help in distinguishing it (refer Sect. 3 in chapter "Imaging of Otomastoiditis, Acute and Chronic").

Further Reading

Booth TN, Vezina LG, Karcher G, Dubovsky EC (2000) Imaging and clinical evaluation of isolated atresia of the oval window. AJNR Am J Neuroradiol 21(1):171–174

Zeifer B, Sabini P, Sonne J (2000) Congenital absence of the oval window: radiologic diagnosis and associated anomalies. AJNR Am J Neuroradiol 21(2):322–327

Congenital Abnormalities of the Inner Ear

Lin Wah Goh and Thi Nguyen

Contents

L. W. Goh (✉)
Department of Diagnostic Radiology, Khoo Teck
Puat Hospital, Singapore, Singapore
e-mail: goh.lin.wah@ktph.com.sg

T. Nguyen
Benson Radiology, Adelaide, Australia
e-mail: thi.nguyen@bensonradiology.com.au

Abstract

This chapter lays out a simplified overview of congenital inner ear abnormalities. A brief description of the inner ear embryology and different classifications is given to impart the reader with a better understanding of the pathology behind the common inner ear malformations. A diagnostic approach is formulated to ensure a practical and surgically relevant report. Each condition is illustrated with pertinent examples.

© Springer Nature Switzerland AG 2021
G. G. Pulickal et al. (eds.), *Temporal Bone Imaging Made Easy*,
Medical Radiology Diagnostic Imaging, https://doi.org/10.1007/978-3-030-70635-7_15

1 Introduction and Basic Embryology

Congenital sensorineural hearing loss is a common cause of disability in newborns worldwide; causes may be genetic or nongenetic. Genetic causes, both syndromic (e.g. CHARGE, Pendred or Alport syndromes etc.) and nonsyndromic, account for about half the cases, with nonsyndromic cases (autosomal dominant or recessive) making up the bulk. Nongenetic causes account for the other half of cases and include intrauterine infection, birth injuries, or environmental causes.

In the third gestational week, otic placodes arise along the lateral surfaces of the neural tube. These placodes eventually invaginate in the fourth gestational week to form a simple cavity called the otocyst. Three primordial folds arise from this cavity by the fifth week, which will eventually develop into the cochlea, vestibule/semicircular canals (SCCs), and endolymphatic sac.

From the fifth gestational week onward, the cochlea undergoes a maturation process that culminates in its complete adult configuration (2.5 turns) by the eighth gestational week. The SCCs start developing from the rudimentary vestibule by the sixth week, beginning with the superior, followed by the posterior, and finally the lateral semicircular canal. The vestibular aqueduct begins its embryological journey as an enlarged cavity that slowly narrows in size from the fifth to eighth week. The entire evolution of the inner ear completes only by the 26th week.

Classifications of congenital inner ear abnormalities are largely based on the works of Jackler et al. in 1987, which tried to classify anomalies based on the timelines of inner ear embryogenesis. The subsequent revisions proposed by Sennaroglu et al. in 2002 who with the aid of modern cross-sectional imaging classified the anomalies on the severity degree of malformation and further subclassified incomplete partition.

2 Choice of Imaging

Cross-sectional imaging is used for a variety of reasons in newborns with sensorineural hearing loss; to establish cause, presurgical assessment of temporal bone anatomy, or auditory pathway and to look for malformations that may predict further progression of hearing loss (prognostication).

Despite the radiation burden, CT remains the preferred modality of choice in most centers, given its widespread availability and quickness in performing the study. CT allows for accurate preoperative assessment of the bony anatomy, inner ear malformations as well as the middle ear cavity and external ear.

While MR imaging without ionizing radiation is attractive, the longer acquisition time, need for sedation, and potential necessity for a preoperative CT anyway can make it a difficult study to justify.

In some instances, e.g., in precochlear implant assessment of the cochlear nerve with heavy T2-weighted 3D sequences is far superior to conventional CT, where often the hypoplasia/aplasia can only be inferred by secondary signs such as the caliber of the cochlear nerve canal (average width of the cochlear nerve canal on CT axial plane is about 1.7 mm) or IAC, which is not reliable.

3 Approach to Congenital Inner Ear Lesions

While reporting a study with congenital inner ear anomalies, it is important to remember that the idea behind imaging is not only diagnosis but also to determine whether the patient would benefit from a hearing device, i.e., cochlear implant. Gross malformations are contraindicative (e.g., Michel or cochlea aplasia), whereas major malformations place the patient at higher risk for surgical complications.

Depending on how early the developmental insult occurs, the more profound the

Table 1 Common congenital inner ear lesions

Condition	Major features	IAC	CN VIII	CN VII	Vestibular aqueduct
Michel Aplasia	• Complete labyrinthine absence	Hypoplastic	Absent	Anomalous	Absent
Cochlea aplasia	• Aplastic cochlea and cochlear nerve canal • Rest of inner ear structures variable	Hypoplastic	Absent	Anomalous	Normal
Common cavity	• "Fused" cochlea and vestibule	Variable	Hypoplastic or absent	Anomalous	Absent
Type 1 Incomplete Partition	• Cystic cochlea and absent modiolus • Varying degrees of vestibule and SCC dysplasia	Widened	Hypoplastic or absent	Variable	Normal
Cochlear hypoplasia	• Underdeveloped cochlea	Variable	Hypoplastic or absent	Aberrant	Variable
Type 2 Incomplete Partition	• Bulbous middle turn and apex with spared basal turn of cochlea	Normal	Normal	Normal	Dilated
Type 3 Incomplete partition	• Corkscrew cochlea • Loss of cribriform plate	Widened (bulbous)	Normal	Aberrant	Variable

malformation is bound to be. Hence, approach the problem from the spectrum of most severe malformations to mild anomalies, i.e., check whether the bony otic capsule is formed at all and then work yourself forward. Are you able to differentiate the individual inner ear components (cochlea, vestibule, SCC, and vestibular aqueduct), and if yes how close to normal do these structures appear to be?

Try to assess the status of the cochlear nerve (as discussed, the degree of confidence depends on the imaging modality), since severe hypoplasia/aplasia is generally contraindicative to implant insertion. Comment upon the caliber of the IAC; is it normal, widened, or hypoplastic? A widened IAC makes the patient more susceptible to postoperative meningitis or gusher. Also comment on the middle ear and ossicles, which are usually normal but stapes malformation and oval window atresia can be seen occasionally.

Remember that most congenital anomalies can be unilateral or bilateral and if bilateral then usually asymmetric (mention which side has worse malformations). Do note that a vast number of these cases may not have any discernable radiological abnormality at all if the insult happened during the maturation stage rather than the developmental phase. The most common cochlear anomalies have been summarized below (Table 1).

4 Complete Labyrinthine Aplasia (Michel Aplasia)

This rare anomaly occurs when the labyrinth fails to develop in the third gestational week and is defined by the complete absence of the cochlea, vestibule, and semicircular canals (SCC) (Fig. 1). The otic capsule bone and petrous apex may be completely absent or severely hypoplastic with a single or several cystic cavities being noted instead. The IAC will be hypoplastic and the vestibulocochlear nerve absent, with the facial nerve having an anomalous course. Absence of a normal oval and round window will result in varying dysplastic changes in the middle ear structures as well.

Usually, this condition does not pose a significant diagnostic challenge with the possible exception being severe labyrinthitis ossificans. Appreciation of a normal amount of otic capsule bone with a well-defined cochlear promontory (formed by the cochlea basal turn) as well as a normal ipsilateral IAC allows for differentiation from severe labyrinthitis ossificans.

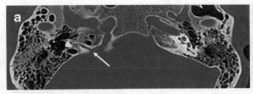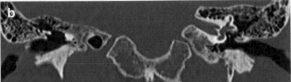

Fig. 1 (a and b) Axial (a) and coronal (b) CT images of a patient with profound right-sided hearing loss shows complete aplasia of the right otic capsule with absence of the cochlea, vestibule, and semicircular canals. The

petrous apex and the internal acoustic meatus are hypoplastic as well (arrow), and the cochlear promontory is not formed. Note the contralateral normal side for comparison

5 Cochlear Aplasia

This rare condition occurs due to arrested development during the early part of fifth gestational week; absence of the cochlea and cochlear nerve canal are the hallmarks of this condition (Fig. 2).

The appearance of the rest of the inner structures is variable; the vestibule and SCCs may be normal or malformed, appearing dilated, globular, or hypoplastic. The internal acoustic meatus (IAM) is usually hypoplastic, and the facial nerve canal takes an anomalous course. The vestibular aqueduct usually remains normal.

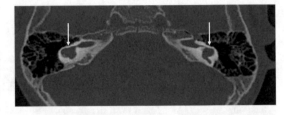

Fig. 2 Axial CT image of a child with bilateral hearing loss shows absence of the cochlea bilaterally and globular malformations of the vestibuli (arrows)

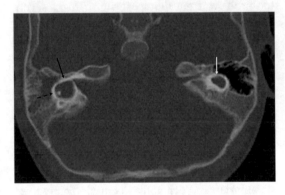

6 Common Cavity

Developmental arrest in the fourth week leads to this condition in which the undifferentiated cochlea and vestibule are still fused into a single "common cavity" (Fig. 3), where individual components of the labyrinth cannot be singled out. The size of the cavity is variable, and the SCC may be absent, malformed, or normal in appearance.

The IAM can have a variable appearance, and the facial nerve canal takes an anomalous course. The vestibular aqueduct may be absent.

7 Type 1 Incomplete Partition (IP-1)

This condition is also known as cystic cochleovestibular malformation (CCVM) and occurs due to arrested development of the otic placode in the fifth gestational week. The hallmarks of this

Fig. 3 Axial CT image of a child with hearing loss shows common cavity deformity on the left side (white arrow) and a narrowed left IAC. There are other anomalies on the right side, with a dilated vestibule (black arrow) and shortened dysplastic lateral semicircular canal (dashed black arrow)

condition are the lack of interscalar septum, and absent modiolus leading to a cystic appearance of the cochlea, the vestibule still can be appreciated separately from the cochlea as opposed to the common cavity deformity described earlier.

Varying degrees of severity depend on the extent of associated vestibule and SCC abnormalities, with the most severe form manifesting as a dilated vestibule and lateral SCC with a cystic cochlear cavity (Fig. 4). The IAM is

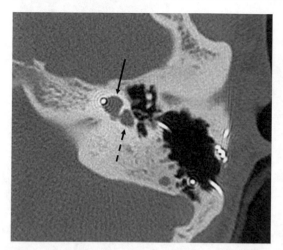

Fig. 4 Axial CT image of a patient with known type 1 incomplete partition, postcochlear implant surgery. Note the lack of internal septation within the cochlea and absent modiolus (arrow) and the separate dilated vestibule and lateral SCC (dashed arrow) forming the classical "Figure 8" appearance (an electrode of cochlear implant could be seen within the cystic cochlea)

usually widened, and the vestibular aqueduct is normal.

Tip

The common cavity, cystic cochleovestibular malformation (IP-1), or cochlear aplasia (especially with globular malformation of the vestibule and SCC) can often be mistaken for each other.

- *Cochlea aplasia is associated with a hypoplastic IAC, whereas IP-1 has usually a widened IAC and the IAC can be variable in common cavity malformation.*
- *If the lateral semicircular canal is incorporated into the cystic cavity, and the vestibule and cochlea cannot be appreciated separately, then common cavity is more likely.*
- *If the large cystic structure appears more like two separate featureless cystic spaces and some degree of separation is still possible (like a figure of eight); then CCVM is favored.*

8 Cochlear Hypoplasia

This condition occurs when the developmental disruption happens in the sixth week of gestation. The cochlea and vestibule are separated, but the cochlea is underdeveloped with less than two turns being present.

The spectrum of severity can range considerably (Figs. 5 and 6) from a simple rudimentary cochlea bud to a cochlea with intact internal architecture/modiolus but with reduced size.

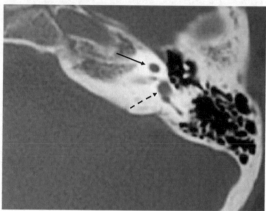

Fig. 5 Axial CT image of a patient with cochlea hypoplasia shows the cochlea as a rudimentary small bud (arrow). The vestibule (dashed arrow) appears to be slightly hypoplastic as well

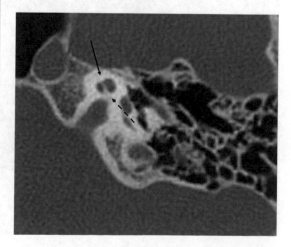

Fig. 6 Axial CT image of another patient with cochlear hypoplasia shows a slightly better formed cochlea (though still less than 2 turns) (arrow) with an absent cochlear nerve canal (dashed arrow)

The cochlea nerve is usually hypoplastic or absent.

The appearance of the rest of the inner ear structures (IAM, cochlea nerve canal, SCC, vestibular aqueduct, etc.) can differ considerably from normal to dysplasia of varying degrees.

9 Type 2 Incomplete Partition (IP-2)

This is the most common inner ear malformation and probably occurs when the developmental arrest occurs late in the seventh gestational week. IP-2 occurs when there is incomplete partitioning between the middle and apical turns of the cochlea due to the absence of the inter scalar septum. This results in a bulbous middle turn/apex with a spared normal basal turn (overall less than 2 turns) and a dysplastic (or absent) modiolus (Fig. 7).

The appearance of the vestibule is variable (normal or dilated), but there is a strong association with a dilated vestibular aqueduct and endolymphatic sac.

The historical term Mondini anomaly has been loosely used by clinicians and radiologists alike, leading to a great deal of confusion. The original report published in 1791 by Carlo Mondini in Latin described a condition in which the cochlea was abnormal having only 1.5 turns with a normal basal turn and cystic apex, an enlarged vestibule but without any accompanying SCCs dysplasia, and an enlarged vestibular aqueduct with dilated endolymphatic sac. Only if this triad of findings is present should the term "Mondini anomaly/deformity or dysplasia" be applied and not elsewhere.

> **Tip**
> • *The absent interscalar septum is associated with a dysplastic osseous spiral lamina that can mimic the interscalar septum on MR imaging and hence confirm on CT.*

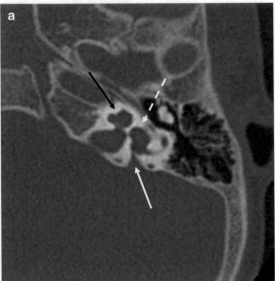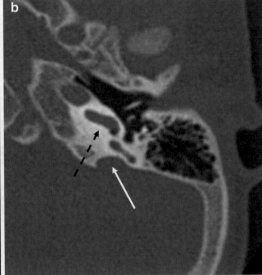

Fig. 7 (**a** and **b**) Contiguous axial CT images of the same patient show a classical Mondini dysplasia depicting an abnormal bulbous middle and apical turns of the cochlea (black arrow) but with a preserved basal turn (dashed black arrow), enlarged vestibular aqueduct (white arrows), and a mildly enlarged vestibule (dashed white arrow) with grossly normal-appearing SCCs

10   Type 3 Incomplete Partition (IP-3)

This is an X-linked recessive disease and usually results in mixed sensorineural and equivocal conductive hearing loss in male patients, with female carriers having normal hearing or minimal loss only.

In IP-3, there is complete loss of the inter scalar septum resulting in a classical "corkscrew" appearance of the cochlea and absence of the modiolus (Fig. 8). The appearance of the vestibule, SCC, and vestibular aqueduct is variable and may be normal or slightly dilated with possible ossification in the SCC. The conductive hearing loss element may be due to stapes footplate fixation.

Another important imaging feature is the widening of the IAM fundus (bilateral and symmetrical) and loss of the cribriform plate that lies between the basal turn of the cochlea and the IAM fundus. This finding is important, as it brings the perilymph in the cochlea and CSF in the IAM in close contact with each other and could result in perilymphatic hydrops or gusher if stapedectomy is attempted. These patients are also at high risk of meningitis, labyrinthitis ossificans, and inadvertent electrode displacement into the IAC during cochlear implant insertion.

11   Malformations of the Semicircular Canals

The SCC can be dysplastic (hypoplasia or enlargement) or be completely absent (aplasia), with dysplasia being far more common.

The most common abnormality being fusion of the dysplastic lateral SCC with the vestibule (which can be dilated or normal) (Fig. 9), the bone island between the SCC, and vestibule is usually very small or completely absent. Abnormality of the lateral semicircular canal can occur in isolation, since it is the last SCC to be formed embryologically. Hypoplasia of all the SCC and the vestibule is suggestive of CHARGE syndrome.

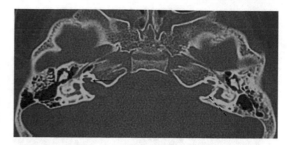

Fig. 8 Axial CT image a patient with type 3 incomplete partition shows loss of cribriform plate (arrow) between the basal turn of the dysplastic cochlea and the symmetrically widened IAM fundi (dashed arrow)

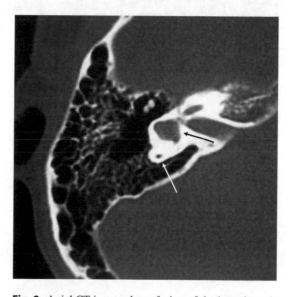

Fig. 9 Axial CT image shows fusion of the lateral semicircular canal and an enlarged vestibule (black arrow), the small bony island usually seen between these structures is absent in this case. The partly visualized posterior semicircular canal (white arrow) appears to be normal

12   Enlarged Vestibular Aqueduct Syndrome (EVAS)

EVAS is the most commonly identified abnormality in patients with early-onset SNHL. It is bilateral in up to 90% of cases and associated with other inner ear anomalies in up to 84% including cochlear anomalies, and dysplasia of the semicircular canals. EVAS is frequently seen in Pendred syndrome, characterized by congenital SNHL, and thyroid goiter.

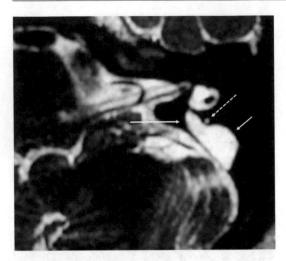

Fig. 10 Axial T2 MR image shows a dilated right vestibular aqueduct (long arrow) and endolymphatic sac (short arrow), note the adjacent normal caliber posterior semicircular canal for comparison (dashed arrow)

Patients present with progressive, early-onset SNHL. Disease progression may also be precipitated by head trauma, changes in barometric pressure, or raised intracranial pressure.

EVAS is best depicted on MR with thin section heavily T2-weighted sequences. The vestibular aqueduct is enlarged when its midpoint measures >0.9 mm or its operculum >1.9 mm (Cincinnati criteria). A simple rule is to compare the diameter of the vestibular aqueduct to the posterior semicircular canal—if larger, it is likely to be abnormal (Fig. 10).

Further Reading

Casselman JW, Offeciers EF, De Foer B, Govaerts P, Kuhweide R, Somers T (2001) CT and MR imaging of congenital abnormalities of the inner ear and internal auditory canal. Eur J Radiol 40:94–104

Huang BY, Zdanski C, Castillo M (2012) Pediatric sensorineural hearing loss, part 1: practical aspects for neuroradiologists. Am J Neuroradiol 33:211–217. https://doi.org/10.3174/ajnr.A2498

Joshi VM, Navlekar SK, Kishore GR, Reddy KJ, Kumar EC (2012) CT and MR imaging of the inner ear and brain in children with congenital sensorineural hearing loss. Radiographics 32:683–698. https://doi.org/10.1148/rg.323115073

Lo WW (1999) What is a 'Mondini' and what difference does a name make? AJNR Am J Neuroradiol 20(8):1442–1444

Vijayasekaran S, Halsted MJ, Boston M, Meinzen-Derr J, Bardo DM, Greinwald J, Benton C (2007) When is the vestibular aqueduct enlarged? A statistical analysis of the normative distribution of vestibular aqueduct size. Am J Neuroradiol 28(6):1133–1138

Yiin RS, Tang PH, Tan TY (2011) Review of congenital inner ear abnormalities on CT temporal bone. Br J of Radiol 84:859–863. https://doi.org/10.1259/bjr/18998800

Radiological Features of Otosclerosis

Geoiphy George Pulickal

Contents

Abstract

This chapter provides an overview of the clinical and radiological features of otosclerosis. All important radiological features are highlighted with appropriate imaging examples. Potential differential diagnosis and pitfalls are explained along with a detailed surgical checklist highlighting the relevant points that need to be included in a practical report.

1 What Is Otosclerosis (or Otospongiosis)

Otosclerosis is an idiopathic (familial or sporadic) bone disease characterized by faulty bone remodelling affecting the otic capsule. Bone is initially resorbed (spongiosis) and then replaced by new aberrant bone (sclerosis). Thus, the term 'otosclerosis' is rather misleading and incomplete. This condition is challenging to diagnose on imaging in the absence of adequate clinical information.

2 Classification

Otosclerosis is divided into two types, fenestral (Fig. 1) and retrofenestral (Fig. 2) disease, with the latter almost always co-existing with the former.

G. G. Pulickal (✉)
Department of Diagnostic Radiology, Khoo Teck Puat Hospital, Singapore, Singapore
e-mail: pulickal.george.geoiphy@ktph.com.sg

© Springer Nature Switzerland AG 2021
G. G. Pulickal et al. (eds.), *Temporal Bone Imaging Made Easy*,
Medical Radiology Diagnostic Imaging, https://doi.org/10.1007/978-3-030-70635-7_16

In fenestral otosclerosis, the pathology involves the lateral wall of the otic capsule, most commonly in and around the fissula ante fenestram and hence the name 'fenestral disease'. The fissula is a cleft of fibrocartilaginous tissue located just anterior to the oval window. Other potential sites for this subtype include the round window, promontory and facial nerve canal.

In retro-fenestral disease, there is involvement of the cochlear capsule, and invariably there will be advanced fenestral disease as well. The lesions can also be seen along the IAC, vestibule and the semi-circular canals.

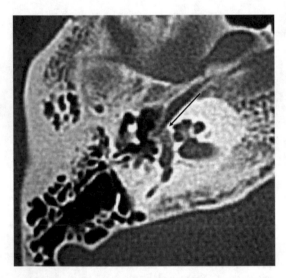

Fig. 1 Axial CT image of a patient with right-sided CHL shows hypodense spongiotic plaque at the fissula ante fenestram

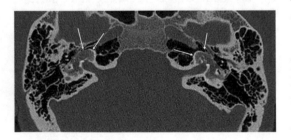

Fig. 2 Axial CT image shows profound bilateral retrofenestral otosclerosis with a thick ring-like otospongiotic plaques around the barely visible cochlea (arrows). Note that the fissula ante-fenestram is involved bilaterally as well

Tip
- *Another type of otospongiosis is the 'cavitary subtype' (Fig. 3), where low-density lesions in the shapes of well-defined notches or diverticula are seen along the anteroinferior aspect of the IAC (Fig. 3), predominantly in elderly patients. Although they have been implicated in third-window phenomenon, sensorineural hearing loss and poorer surgical outcomes, these claims remain controversial for now.*

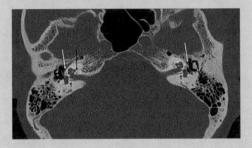

Fig. 3 Axial CT image of an elderly patient with bilateral hearing loss show otospongiotic plaques in bilateral fissula ante-fenestram (white arrows), more prominent on the left. Note the bud-like hypodensity along the anterior margin of the IAC consistent with a cavitary lesion (black arrow). This lesion is not to be mistaken with the normal singular canal (dashed black arrows) along the posterior margin of the IAC

3   Clinical Features and Management

Patients usually present with conductive hearing loss (CHL) (fenestral type), although sensorineural and mixed hearing loss can occur in advanced disease (retro-fenestral involvement). The pathology tends to be bilateral (85%), worldwide in distribution and with a clear female preponderance.

Audiogram shows a classical 'Carhart notch', which is a characteristic dip in the bone conduction audiogram at 2000 Hz. On otoscopy, hyper-aemia of the cochlear promontory is sometimes observed, referred to as 'Schwarze Sign' (in ret-rofenestral disease).

Treatment is usually surgical through sta-pedotomy or stapedectomy and prosthesis inser-tion. Severe retrofenestral disease may benefit from cochlea implantation.

4 Choice of Imaging and Imaging Features

CT of the temporal bone using 1-mm (or less)-thick sections with multiplanar reconstructions is the modality of choice. MRI has only a limited role, other than in planning for possible hearing aid implantation, e.g. to check for calibre/pres-ence of the cochlear nerve.

The imaging features mirror the bone remod-elling process with 'hypodense plaques' seen in the spongiotic phase and 'heaped-up' aberrant bone in the sclerotic phase.

The otic capsule is usually homogenously dense, and any lucency encountered in the typical locations, i.e. at the fissula, around the oval/round windows and cochlea should be deemed suspi-cious (Fig. 4). The plaques can have a wide range of appearance from being extremely subtle and hazy to large and conspicuous.

Classically in the sclerotic phase, heaped-up bone can be seen encroaching upon the oval win-dow (sometimes obliterating it) and the stapes footplate (Fig. 5). This can cause fixation of the stapes-vestibular joint giving rise to the charac-teristic CHL encountered in this condition; hence, these structures should be carefully inspected on multiple planes.

Retro-fenestral disease shows involvement beyond the fissula with the peri-cochlear regions being affected. Classically, a hypodense 'halo' forms around the cochlea which is termed the fourth ring of Valvassori (the basal, middle and apical turns of the cochlea being the normal three rings). If imaging is done in the sclerotic phase and no contour distorting "heaped-up bone" is present, then imaging can be falsely normal at times.

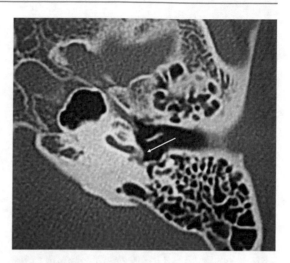

Fig. 4 Axial CT image shows an otospongiotic plaque involving the round window (arrow) and completely oblit-erating it

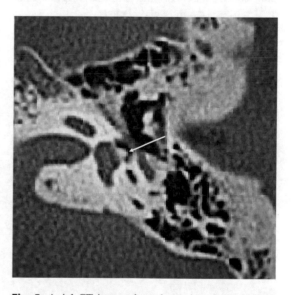

Fig. 5 Axial CT image shows heaped up bone (arrow) over the oval window completely covering it, finding is compatible with otosclerosis. Note the absence of any hypodense spongiotic plaques

5 Differentials

The most important differential for otosclerosis is the 'cochlear cleft', which is a normal anatomi-cal non-osseous space in the region of the fissula ante fenestram. It is more commonly seen in childhood and becomes less frequent with advancing age. It appears as a well-defined

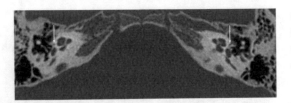

Fig. 6 Axial CT image shows incidental bilateral symmetrical tiny hypodensities in the fissual ante fenestram (arrow), compatible with cochlear clefts

symmetrical CT hypodensity that is small and round on axial planes and thin and curvilinear on coronal planes. It lies lateral to the middle turn of the cochlea but does not 'touch' it (Fig. 6) and also does not extend to the anterior margin of the oval window on the axial plane. True otospongiotic plaques are broader and usually less well-defined and extend to the anterior margin of the oval window on the axial plane.

Advanced otosclerosis can sometimes be mistaken with other bone diseases such as Pagets disease (shows skull involvement beyond the temporal bones) and osteogenesis imperfecta (systemic involvement), but this is usually not a diagnostic dilemma.

> **Tip**
> - *Utilize multiplanar reformations with localizer to confirm the presence of plaques if lesions appear equivocal on conventional projections.*
> - *Avoid 'satisfaction of search' and don't overlook mild disease on asymptomatic side.*

6 What the Surgeon Wants to Know

> **Surgical Checklist**
> - Could the hearing loss be due to other diseases which may present clinically like otosclerosis, e.g. congenital oval window atresia, ossicular discontinuity/fixation, dehiscence of superior semicircular canal etc.?
> - Type of otosclerosis, fenestral or retrofenestral disease, as this will determine the type of treatment.
> - Check for bilateral disease, symptoms may be unilateral, but pathology is *commonly bilateral.*
> - Which side is more severely affected? Assessed by the thickening of the stapes footplate in the axial plane and the height of the oval window in the coronal plane; the normal height is about 2 mm.
> - Are the oval or round windows involved, if yes still patent or obliterated?
> - What is the status of the facial nerve canal, is there any focal dehiscence with protrusion? If yes, to what degree does the protruded nerve cover the oval window? (Fig. 7)
> - Are there any concomitant inner ear anomalies? As this raises the possibility of increased pressure in the inner ear and puts the patient at an increased risk of gusher during stapedotomy.

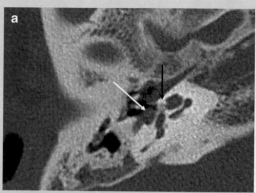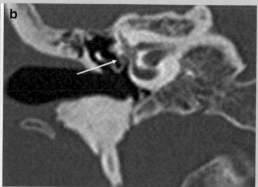

Fig. 7 Axial and coronal CT images of a patient with right-sided CHL show a spongiotic plaque at the fissual ante fenestram (black arrow). Note the protruded tympanic segment of the facial nerve completely covering the oval window (white arrows)

Further Reading

Puac P, Rodríguez A, Lin HC, Onofrj V, Lin FC, Hung SC, Zamora C, Castillo M (2018) Cavitary plaques in otospongiosis: CT findings and clinical implications. AJNR Am J Neuroradiol 39(6):1135–1139. https://doi.org/10.3174/ajnr.A5613. Epub 2018 Apr 5

Purohit B, Hermans R (2014) Op de Beeck K. Imaging in otosclerosis: a pictorial review. Insights Imaging 5(2):245–252. https://doi.org/10.1007/s13244-014-0313-9. Epub 2014 Feb 9

Valvassori GE (1993) Imaging of otosclerosis. Otolaryngol Clin N Am 26(3):359–371

Other Causes of Inner Ear Hearing Loss: Meniere's Disease, Labyrinthitis and Semi-Circular Canal Dehiscence

Thi Nguyen and Filipe Vilas Boas

Contents

Abstract

This chapter provides an overview of a few miscellaneous inner ear conditions that could give rise to hearing loss. The pathophysiology, clinical and radiological features of Meniere's disease are detailed with illustrative cases provided for each grade. Labyrinthitis and its potential mimics are discussed, and a differentiating table is given for easy reference. Finally, semi-circular canal dehiscence is outlined with a guide on imaging reformations and few examples.

T. Nguyen (✉)
Benson Radiology, Adelaide, Australia
e-mail: thi.nguyen@bensonradiology.com.au

F. V. Boas
Royal Adelaide Hospital, Adelaide, Australia
e-mail: Filipe.vilasboas@sa.gov.au

1 Meniere's Disease

1.1 What Is Meniere's Disease

Meniere's disease (MD) is a clinical syndrome secondary to altered inner ear fluid homeostasis causing spontaneous episodes of vertigo, fluctuating hearing loss, aural fullness, and

© Springer Nature Switzerland AG 2021
G. G. Pulickal et al. (eds.), *Temporal Bone Imaging Made Easy*,
Medical Radiology Diagnostic Imaging, https://doi.org/10.1007/978-3-030-70635-7_17

tinnitus. A characteristic pathologic feature of MD is endolymphatic hydrops (EH) which is an excessive accumulation of endolymph in the vestibule and cochlea. Although not all patients with EH have MD, its cause and relationship remain unclear.

1.2 Clinical Features and Management

One or both ears can be affected, and symptoms usually present in middle-aged patients. As per the American Academy of Otolaryngology-Head and Neck Surgery Committee on Hearing and Equilibrium (revised in 2015), the criteria for the diagnosis of MD are divided into definite and probable.

Definite criteria include two or more episodes of vertigo lasting 20 min to 12 h, audiometry-confirmed low-medium frequency hearing loss and fluctuating aural symptoms (hearing, tinnitus or fullness) in the affected ear, all of which are not better accounted for by another diagnosis.

In most patients, the clinical symptoms of MD manifest after significant accumulation of endolymph. Vertiginous symptoms in MD are multifactorial in their aetiology but are believed to stem from leakage of high-potassium endolymph into the perilymph compartment. Hearing loss stems from distension of the basilar membrane (involved in sound transmission and amplification), impairing its function. The basilar membrane is softer and more pliable at the cochlear apex, which is responsible for low-frequency sound transmission, and thus patients classically present initially with low-frequency hearing loss.

Management is targeted at providing relief during acute attacks and preventing progressive damage to hearing and vestibular function. Treatment approach to MD is divided into medical and surgical interventions. Intra-tympanic steroid therapy has long been used due to the proposed inflammatory component of MD and postulated permeability of steroids through the blood-labyrinth barrier reaching the perilymphatic compartment. Ablative therapies using intra-tympanic Gentamicin works due to the vestibulotoxic effects; however, the associated ototoxic effects (damage to hair cells and subsequent hearing loss) are a major disadvantage. Rarely, in cases refractory to medical management, surgical interventions are considered such as surgical labyrinthectomy and vestibular neurotomy.

1.3 Choice of Imaging

The idea behind imaging in MD can be twofold, to exclude any other possible cause for the symptoms (e.g. vestibular Schwannoma, neurovascular conflict etc.) or to demonstrate endolymphatic hydrops. MR imaging is the modality of choice in both instances.

Imaging for endolymphatic hydrops is an evolving science with significant advances occurring this past decade. It is performed with a 3 T magnet utilising a heavily T2-weighted 3D-FLAIR sequence 4 h post-intravenous gadolinium injection.

Endolymph and perilymph compartments are indistinguishable from each other on routine non-contrast sequences. The post-gadolinium 3D-FLAIR sequences allow discrimination between these compartments because gadolinium can accumulate within the perilymphatic space appearing as bright signal, outlining the endolymphatic compartment which is impermeable to contrast and appears as a filling defect. Subtraction and reversal images can then be obtained from these images to enhance the discrimination between the endo/perilymph, from adjacent bone and air, to further increase specificity.

1.4 Imaging Features

EH is assessed on high-resolution axial 3D-FLAIR post-gadolinium sequences. Several grading systems have been utilised, with Bernaerts et al. recently proposing a 2-point scoring system for cochlear hydrops and 3-point system for vestibular hydrops (Table 1).

Assessment for vestibular hydrops (VH) requires evaluation of the saccule (found

Table 1 Grading for cochlear and vestibular hydrops

	Cochlear	Vestibular
Grade 1 hydrops	Nodular dilation of the cochlear duct	Inversion of the saccule/utricle ratio without conglomeration
Grade 2 hydrops	Diffuse distension of the cochlear duct with Scala vestibuli effacement	Dilation of saccule/utricle involving >50% of the vestibule
Grade 3 hydrops		Complete obliteration of vestibular perilymphatic signal by dilated saccule/utricle

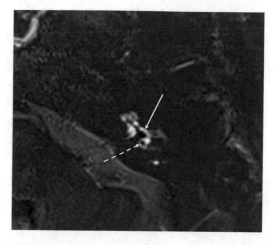

Fig. 2 Axial MR post-contrast 3D FLAIR image shows an inverted saccule–utricle ratio with a dilated saccule (arrow) and a separate normal-sized utricle (dashed arrow), consistent with grade 1 VH

anteroinferiorly within the vestibule) and utricle (found posterosuperiorly). In the normal setting, the utricle and saccule appear as two discrete punctate structures (Fig. 1). Grade 1 VH is characterised by preferential enlargement of the saccule, equal to or larger than the utricle, but without conglomeration (saccule-utricle-ratio-inversion) (Fig. 2). Grade 2 VH results when the utricle and saccule conglomerate and occupy greater than 50% of the vestibule (Fig. 3). Grade 3 VH is characterised by enlargement of the utricle/saccule causing complete effacement of the vestibular perilymph (Fig. 4).

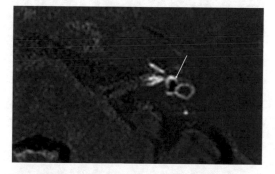

Fig. 3 Axial MR post-contrast 3D FLAIR image shows a confluent saccule and utricle occupying more than half of the vestibule (arrow), consistent with grade 2 VH

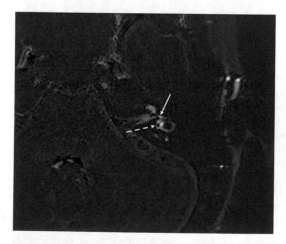

Fig. 1 Axial MR post-contrast 3D FLAIR image shows the normal saccule (arrow) and utricle (dashed arrow) as two distinctly separate small hypodensities within the vestibule

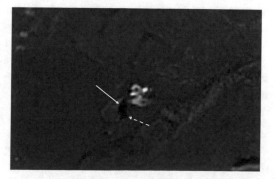

Fig. 4 Axial MR post-contrast 3D FLAIR image shows almost complete obliteration of the vestibule with barely any peri-lymphatic enhancement being visible (arrow). Note how the dilated utricle begins to protrude through the lateral semi-circular canal (dashed arrow), consistent with grade 3 VH

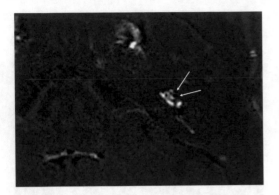

Fig. 5 Axial MR post-contrast 3D FLAIR image shows focal-filling defects in the Scala vestibuli by the dilated Scala media (arrows) consistent with grade 1 CH

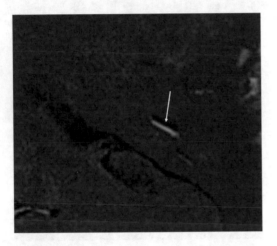

Fig. 6 Axial MR post-contrast 3D FLAIR image shows complete obliteration of the Scala vestibuli by the enlarged Scala media (arrow) consistent with grade 2 CH

Assessment of cochlear hydrops (CH) involves assessment of the cochlear duct/Scala media for enlargement. Grade 1 CH includes nodular dilatation of the Scala media (Fig. 5), while grade 2 CH manifests as diffuse enlargement of the scala media resulting in complete effacement of the scala vestibuli throughout the cochlear turns (Fig. 6).

> **Tip**
> • *Perilymphatic hyperenhancement in MD has been validated as an ancillary imaging feature in patients with MD, a result of increased blood-labyrinthine barrier permeability.*

> • *The presence of unilateral perilymphatic hyperenhancement is suggestive of a diagnosis of MD. In cases where enhancement is symmetric bilaterally, the demonstration of EH is crucial and decisive in order to meet criteria for MD.*

2 Labyrinthitis

2.1 What Is Labyrinthitis?

Labyrinthitis is an inflammatory process of the membranous labyrinth with several potential aetiologies. Viral infections including herpes simplex, influenza and Epstein-Barr virus have been implicated and may be systemic or confined to the vestibulo-cochlear apparatus. Bacterial infections may spread from the middle ear or CSF in the setting of otitis media or meningitis, resulting in a secondary labyrinthitis. Other potential causes include trauma or autoimmune disorders.

2.2 Clinical Features and Management

Patients with labyrinthitis may present with sudden-onset dizziness, vertigo, tinnitus and sensorineural hearing loss. In many, the disease is self-limiting; however, a proportion of patients may have long-lasting symptoms. Treatment options include symptomatic relief, oral or intratympanic steroids and treatment of the underlying aetiology, such as the middle ear infection.

Complications of labyrinthitis include labyrinthine ossificans, which most commonly follows suppurative labyrinthitis and is characterised by replacement of the labyrinth, initially with fibrous tissue, and subsequently by ossific material. In cochlear implant candidates, ossification may limit the surgical placement of electrodes, and dense ossification may be a contraindication for cochlear implantation.

2.3   Choice of Imaging

Classically, the role of imaging in suspected labyrinthitis was to exclude other potential causes such as vestibular Schwannoma. Ever-improving MR imaging capabilities and availability has made MRI the investigation of choice and has led to earlier imaging of patients with sudden-onset hearing loss and has made the early changes in labyrinthitis detectable.

Multi-sequential MR imaging with the use of heavily T2-weighted, T1, FLAIR and post-contrast sequences is able to confidently differentiate between inflammation, haemorrhage, and space-occupying lesions in the labyrinth. Judicious use of 3D sequences allows for extremly fine resolution and multiplanar reconstructions.

The role of CT imaging in acute labyrinthitis is limited with only advanced complications such as labyrinthitis ossificans being visible.

2.4   Imaging Features and Differentials

Typically, in acute labyrinthitis the labyrinth will return normal fluid signal on conventional T2 and T1 sequences, with abnormal hyperintensity only being seen on unenhanced FLAIR and post-contrast T1 sequences due to proteinaceous exudate and altered blood-labyrinthine barrier permeability, respectively (Fig. 7).

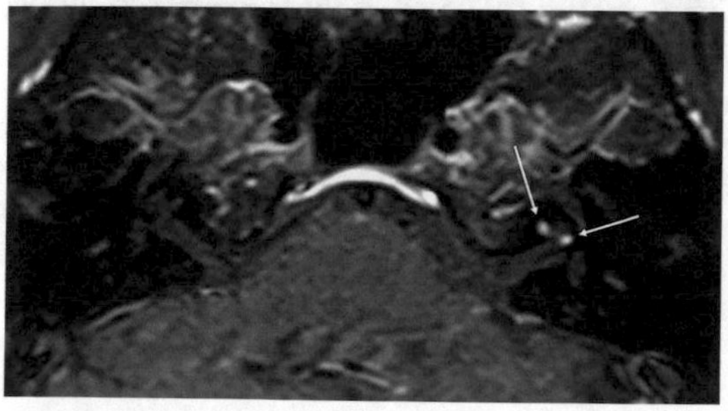

The differential diagnosis of abnormal labyrinthine FLAIR hyperintensity includes intra-labyrinthine haemorrhage, which may present similarly but will also display increased T1 signal differentiating it from labyrinthitis (Fig. 8). With both labyrinthitis and labyrinthine haemorrhage, the normal high signal on heavily T2-weighted sequences may be slightly attenuated, but the labyrinthine outlines remain well defined, and CT imaging of the temporal bones is normal.

In patients who subsequently develop labyrinthine fibrosis, there is loss of the normal high signal on heavily T2-weighted sequences due to fluid replacement by fibrous tissue (Fig. 9). Sometimes some irregularity of the labyrinthine outline and mild residual enhancement can be observed.

This is similar to labyrinthine ossificans on MRI, which also displays loss of T2 signal although the degree of enhancement is further reduced or absent. These conditions can then be distinguished on CT, with labyrinthine ossificans demonstrating replacement of the membranous labyrinth with mature bone formation, whereas for fibrous replacement, the labyrinth would still appear grossly normal.

Intra-labyrinthine schwannomas may also demonstrate some similar imaging features with loss of signal on T2 (appears like a filling defect)

Fig. 7 Axial post-contrast MR image of a patient with acute left-sided sensorineural hearing loss shows patchy enhancement in the left cochlea, consistent with labyrinthitis

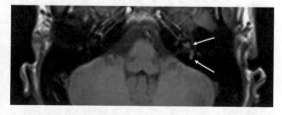

Fig. 8 Axial unenhanced T1 MR image of a patient with known sickle cell anaemia, presenting with acute left-sided sensorineural hearing loss shows T1 hyperintensity in the left cochlea and vestibule. No enhancement was detected on subsequent post-contrast images (not shown). Findings are compatible with labyrinthine haemorrhage. (Courtesy Dr. Ravi Lingam, Northwick Park Hospital, London)

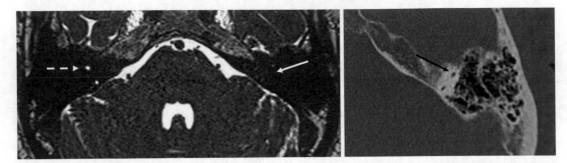

Fig. 9 Axial heavy T2 weight image and corresponding axial CT image of a patient with sensorineural hearing loss show loss of normal fluid signal in the left superior semi-circular canal and almost complete obliteration of its outline (arrow). Note the normal fluid signal on the con-tralateral side (dashed arrow), subsequent CT scan did not show frank ossification of the semi-circular canal (black arrow). Findings indicate labyrinthine fibrosis rather than labyrinthitis ossificans

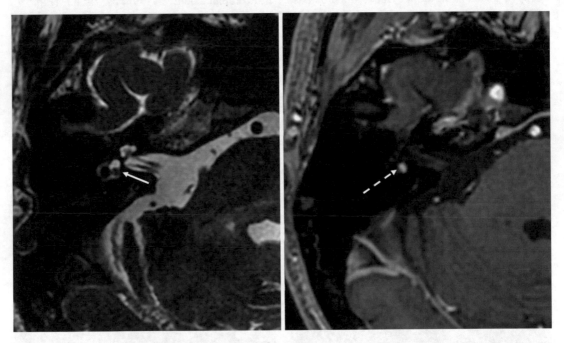

Fig. 10 Axial T2 and post-contrast T1 MR images of a patient with right-sided sensorineural hearing loss, shows a focal hypodense filling defect (arrow) in the vestibule which shows intense focal enhancement. Findings are consistent with an intra-labyrinthine Schwannoma

sequence and subsequent enhancement following contrast administration; however, these are typi-cally more focal rather than diffuse (Fig. 10).

The imaging features of labyrinthitis and potential differential diagnoses are summarised below (Table 2).

Table 2 Imaging features of labyrinthitis and its differential diagnoses

	FLAIR	T1	T2	Post-contrast	CT
Acute labyrinthitis	Increased		Normal or slightly attenuated	Enhances	Normal
Labyrinthine fibrosis	Increased	Increased	Low signal	May show some residual enhancement	Normal
Labyrinthitis ossificans			Low signal	Minimal or no enhancement	Bone formation
Labyrinthine haemorrhage	Increased	Increased	Variable	No enhancement	Normal
Intra-labyrinthine Schwannoma		Hypointense but usually slightly higher signal than CSF	Focal hypo-intensity/ filling defect	Enhancement is focal and avid	Normal, unless lesion is large

3   Semi-circular Canal Dehiscence

3.1   What Is Semi-circular Canal Dehiscence (SCCD)?

SCCD occurs due to a defect in the bony covering of the semi-circular canals resulting in a "third window" effect which in turn results in disordered endolymphatic homeostasis. The aetiology remains uncertain and presumed idiopathic—whilst there may be a congenital or developmental basis in rare cases, it is generally felt to be an acquired disorder.

3.2   Clinical Features and Management

SCCD is characterised by vertigo and nystagmus exacerbated by loud noises (Tullio phenomenon). Other symptoms include oscillopsia, aural fullness, autophony and conductive hearing loss.

Typical audiometric findings include an air-bone gap due to increased bone, and reduced air conduction, typically at lower frequencies (<1 Khz) – a range at which acoustic energy is readily dissipated by the third window effect.

Various surgical treatments including canal resurfacing, capping, plugging or re-enforcement of the oval or round windows (via transmastoid or middle cranial fossa approaches) are used for patient with disabling symptoms.

3.3   Choice of Imaging and Imaging Features

The primary diagnostic imaging test for diagnosis of SCCD is high-resolution CT of the temporal bones, which clearly depicts the bony defects of the canal.

Multiplanar reconstruction is required to prevent partial volume artefacts that could result in false-positive results. SCCD is well depicted in the standard coronal plane, but to further specificity, reformatted oblique images, along the plane of the semicircular canal of the semicircular canal (Poschl view) (Fig. 11) can be acquired.

The superior semi-circular canal is the most frequently involved canal (Fig. 12) followed by the posterior semi-circular canal, which can occur either sporadically or with the superior canal (Fig. 13). Remember to measure the size of the bony dehiscence and describe its exact location.

Occasionally, the possibility of SSSCD may be raised on MRI performed for other indications; however, this should always be correlated with a dedicated CT.

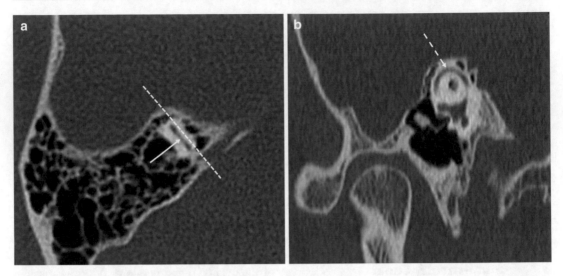

Fig. 11 (**a** and **b**) Axial CT image (**a**) shows the reference slice with the cranial aspect of the superior semicircular canal being seen (arrow). Oblique reconstructions are obtained in the plane parallel to this canal (dashed line). The resultant oblique coronal plane (**b**) will allow for a more complete assessment of superior semi-circular canal and its overlying bony roof (dashed arrow)

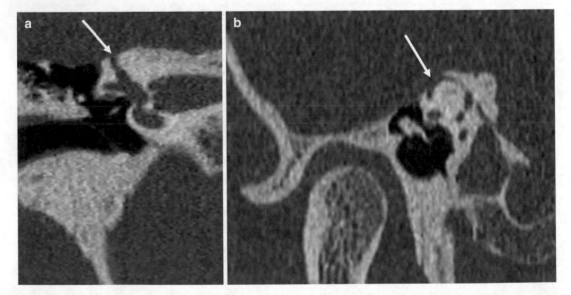

Fig. 12 (**a** and **b**) Conventional CT coronal (**a**) and reformatted Poschl's view (**b**) showing dehiscence of the superior semi-circular canal (arrows) with loss of the normal bony roof covering the semi-circular canal

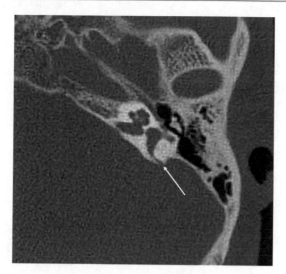

Fig. 13 Axial CT image shows an incidental posterior semi-circular canal dehiscence (arrow)

Further Reading

Bernaerts A, Vanspauwen R, Blaivie C et al (2019) The value of four stage vestibular hydrops grading and asymmetric perilymphatic enhancement in the diagnosis of Meniere's disease on MRI. Neuroradiology 61(4):421–429. https://doi.org/10.1007/s00234-019-02155-7

Conte G, Di Berardino F, Sina C, Zanetti D, Scola E, Gavagna C, Gaini L, Palumbo G, Capaccio P (2017) Triulzi F. MR imaging in sudden sensorineural hearing loss. Time to talk. Am J Neuroradiol 38(8): 1475–1479

Eliezer M, Maquet C, Horion J, Gillibert A, Toupet M, Bolognini B, Magne N, Kahn L, Hautefort C, Attyé A (2019) Detection of intralabyrinthine abnormalities using post-contrast delayed 3D-FLAIR MRI sequences in patients with acute vestibular syndrome. Eur Radiol 29(6):2760–2769

Ho ML, Moonis G, Halpin CF, Curtin HD (2017) Spectrum of third window abnormalities: semicircular canal dehiscence and beyond. Am J Neuroradiol 38(1):2–9

Morimoto K, Yoshida T, Sugiura S et al (2017) Endolymphatic hydrops in patients with unilateral and bilateral Meniere's disease. Acta Otolaryngol 137(1):23–28. https://doi.org/10.1080/00016489.2016.1217042

Nakashima T, Pyykkö I, Arroll MA et al (2016) Meniere's disease. Nat Rev. Dis Primers 2:16028. https://doi.org/10.1038/nrdp.2016.28

van Steekelenburg JM, van Weijnen A, de Pont LMH, Vijlbrief OD, Bommeljé CC, Koopman JP, Verbist BM, Blom HM, Hammer S (2020) Value of endolymphatic hydrops and perilymph signal intensity in suspected Ménière disease. Am J Neuroradiol 41(3):529–534. https://doi.org/10.3174/ajnr.A6410

Part V

Imaging of Temporal Bone Trauma, Petrous Apex, Cerebellopontine Angles, Jugular Foramen and Facial Nerve

Imaging of Temporal Bone Trauma

Pratik Mukherjee

Contents

Abstract

Temporal bone trauma is a frequently encountered clinical issue that requires careful evaluation and precise description in order to exclude serious complications and guide surgical interventions when necessary. This chapter discusses the appropriate trauma imaging strategy based on various clinical settings, reviews the normal anatomy that could potentially mimic fractures, i.e. pseudo-fractures and elaborates on the different types of temporal bone fractures and complications. Quick reference checklists for potential complications, ossicular chain disruptions and important surgical descriptors are provided as well.

P. Mukherjee (✉)
Department of Diagnostic Radiology, Woodlands Health Campus, Singapore, Singapore
e-mail: pratik_mukherjee@whc.sg

1 Pseudo-fractures

The temporal bones are complex paired bony structures that have a myriad of fissures or sutures and are traversed by numerous channels, all of which can potentially be mistaken for fractures.

Fissures that form between the five native parts of the temporal bone are called "intrinsic" and are located around the external ear canal

(EAC). Those fissures that form between the temporal bone and the rest of the skull bones are termed "extrinsic fissures" (Figs. 1 and 2) (Table 1).

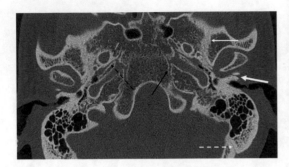

Fig. 1 Axial CT image shows the following extrinsic fissures, i.e. the petro-occipital (black arrow), sphenopetrosal (black dashed arrow), sphenosquamosal (white arrow) and the occipitomastoid (white dashed) fissures as well as the intrinsic tympanosquamous fissure (thick white arrow)

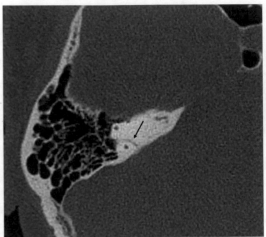

Fig. 3 Axial CT image shows the faint petromastoid canal (arrow) traversing between the anterior and posterior limbs of the superior semi-circular canals, it should always be equal or smaller in calibre than the semi-circular canals

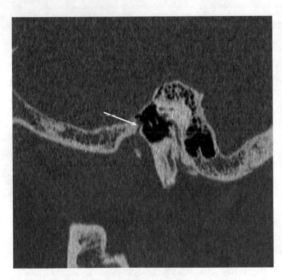

Fig. 2 Sagittal CT shows the petrotympanic fissure (arrow) containing the chorda tympani nerve, extending from the middle ear to the temporomandibular joint

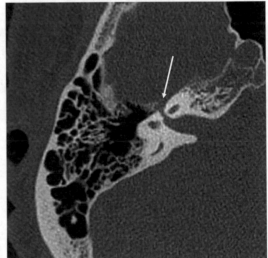

Fig. 4 Axial CT image shows an opening along the anterior surface of the petrous apex that is in continuation with the geniculate ganglion termed the hiatus of the facial nerve, through which the greater superficial petrosal nerve exists

Table 1 Normal fissures and intrinsic channels

Extrinsic fissures	Intrinsic fissures	Intrinsic channels
Sphenosquamosal	Tympanosquamous	Cochlear and vestibular aqueducts (refer Sect. 1 in chapter "Basic Temporal Bone Imaging Anatomy: External, Middle and Inner Ear")
Sphenopetrosal	Petrotympanic	Mastoid and inferior tympanic canaliculi (refer Sect. 5 in chapter "Imaging of the Petrous Apex, Cerebellopontine Angles and Jugular Foramen")
Occipitomastoid	Petrosquamous	Petromastoid (subarcuate) canal (Fig. 3)
Petrooccipital	Tympanomastoid	Hiatus of the facial canal (Fig. 4)
		Singular nerve canal (Fig. 5)

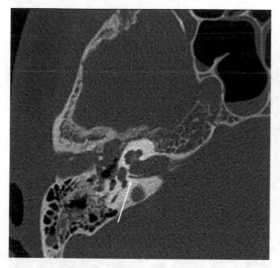

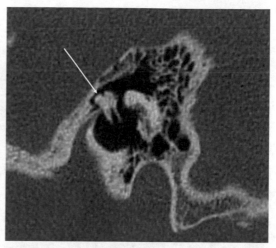

Fig. 5 Axial CT image shows the singular canal (arrow) transmitting the singular nerve from the IAC to the posterior semi-circular canal. Note the post-traumatic changes in the temporal bone with patchy opacifications of the mastoid air cells and EAC

Fig. 6 Oblique CT reconstruction of the malleoincudal joint shows the anteriorly located malleus head (arrow) articulating with the facet of the incus

2 Imaging Approach

High-resolution CT scan with axial fine cuts (preferably sub-1 mm thickness and small field of view i.e. <10 cm) and multiplanar reconstructions is the imaging of choice. Conventional axial and coronal views may not always display the integrity of the ossicular chain adequately; hence, multiplanar reformations (MPR) should be used to overcome this limitation. The idea is to reformat oblique planes in line with the long axis of each individual bone or joint to obtain a holistic view (refer Sect. 1 in chapter "Temporal Bone Imaging Techniques: Computer Tomography, Cone Beam CT and Magnetic Resonance Imaging") (Fig. 6).

> **MRI in Temporal Bone Trauma**
> - MRI has only limited role and should only be used as a problem-solving tool.
> - In persistent post-traumatic vertigo where initial CT evaluation did not show any abnormality, gradient echo sequences can detect haemorrhage

within vestibular nucleus or nerve root entry zone.
- In established CSF otorrhea, high-resolution T2w sequences can detect encephaloceles and pinpoint the exact site of CSF leak. Contrast is useful in such cases to look for dural enhancement which is a secondary sign of dural tear, CSF leak and possible meningitis.
- In post-traumatic facial palsy without any obvious temporal bone fracture, MRI can demonstrate abnormal nerve and dural enhancement along the temporal bone, probably due to tears from micro (occult) fractures

3 Temporal Bone Fractures

Patients with head injury undergo a preliminary CT head in the emergency department, and gross temporal bone fractures are usually readily identifiable. Subtle fractures can be more challenging, and clinicians and radiologists should be aware of some clinical and imaging findings that are suggestive of temporal bone fractures (Table 2).

Table 2 Clinical signs and imaging findings on computed tomography of head which are highly suggestive of temporal bone involvement

Clinical findings suspicious for temporal bone fracture	Indirect imaging signs of temporal bone fracture
Blunt head injury and Racoon eyes (periorbital ecchymosis)	Pneumocephalus adjacent to the temporal bone
	Epidural haematoma (middle meningeal artery injury)
Blood in external auditory canal	Air in the temporomandibular joint (Fig. 7)
Blood in the external ear	Mastoid and/or middle ear opacification (Fig. 7)
Hearing loss, vertigo, imbalance or facial paralysis	Pneumolabyrinth (Fig. 8)

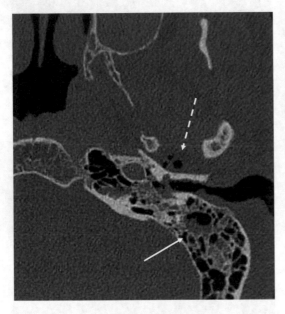

Fig. 7 Axial CT image does not show any obvious temporal bone fracture but air in the temporomandibular joint (dashed arrow) and patchy opacification of the mastoid air cells (arrow) are highly suggestive of a traumatic temporal bone injury

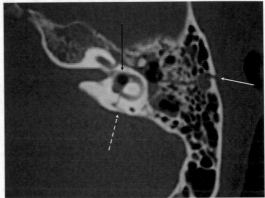

Fig. 8 Axial CT image shows a mixed temporal bone fracture with longitudinal (white arrow) and transverse (dashed arrow) components violating the otic capsule. A focus of pneumolabyrith is seen within the vestibule

Temporal bone fractures are classically divided into longitudinal, transverse and mixed fractures (Table 3) based on the *orientation of the fracture to the petrous segment* of the temporal bone. Unfortunately, this classification does not predict potential complications; hence it is of limited clinical use. Nevertheless, it is still in use as it helps in communicating the findings to the referrer.

Alternatively, more clinical classification systems were developed, e.g. broadly classifying them into petrous and non-petrous or otic-sparing and otic-violating fractures. The otic-violating fractures involve the labyrinth (cochlea, vestibule and semi-circular canals) and are commonly associated with SNHL, CSF fistula and facial nerve injury (Fig. 8). The most popular way is a combined approach, describing the direction of fracture (traditional), location along the temporal bone and involvement of the bony labyrinth/otic capsule (clinical).

Table 3 Review of different types of fractures of temporal bone

Type of fracture	Incidence	Mechanism	Imaging findings

Longitudinal (Fig. 9)	70–90% cases	• Temporo-parietal impact on the head
		• The force being directed laterally to medial along the long axis of the temporal bone
			• Fracture parallel to long axis of petrous segment
			• Fracture can involve EAC, tympanic cavity and squamous segment of temporal bone
			• *Usually spares the inner ear*
			• *Ossicular chain disruptions are more common*
			• Subtypes
			  – Anterior; fracture plane extends anteriorly towards the Eustachian tube and middle cranial fossa (more common)
			  – Posterior; fracture extends behind the bony labyrinth to involve jugular foramen and posterior fossa (rarer)

Transverse	10–20% cases	• Blow to the back or front of the head
		• Force direction is along antero-posterior axis
			• Fracture perpendicular to long axis of petrous segment
			• Subtypes (depending on position of the fracture line relative to arcuate eminence)
			  – Medial; transgresses at or medial to lateral most aspect of internal auditory canal
			  – Lateral; transgresses bony labyrinth

Mixed (Fig. 8)			• Combination of both longitudinal and transverse fractures

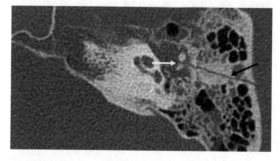

Fig. 9 Axial CT images showing a characteristic otic sparing longitudinal fracture that extends into the middle ear cavity (black arrow) and causes widening/subluxation of the incudomalleolar joint (white arrow)

4 Complications

Temporal bone injuries can give rise to numerous complications; while some like CHL, SNHL and vertigo are rather common, others like otorrhea and facial paralysis are less common. Use the table below as quick reference for the potential causes behind these symptoms (Table 4).

Table 4 Complications of temporal bone trauma based on location and symptoms

Symptoms	Imaging findings
CHL	• Blood in the EAC and Haemotympanum (transient) • TM perforation • Ossicular chain disruption (Figs. 9, 10, 11 and 12)
SNHL and vertigo	• Otic capsule violation • IAC injury • Pneumo or haemolabyrinth (MRI for the latter) → Labyrinthitis ossificans • Nerve root entry zone injury or transection (MRI better)
CSF otorrhea	• Tegmen fracture (Fig. 13) • Stapes footplate-oval window injury • Round window involvement
Facial nerve palsy	• Up to 50% in transverse fractures • Fracture line through the facial nerve canal, usually in the tympanic part. Usually with a bony fragment impinging on the canal (acute) • Post-traumatic oedema or haemorrhage involving facial nerve canal; fracture may be absent (delayed presentation)

Adapted from Kennedy et al. (2014)

Tip
• *Perilymphatic fistula is a rare complication that results due to an abnormal connection between the aerated middle ear and the fluid-filled inner ear.*
• *Patients can present with a variety of symptoms including ear fullness, tinnitus, SNHL, vertigo etc. The site of communication can be the oval or round windows or the otic capsule.*
• *Presence of a middle ear effusion with opacification of the windows or presence of a pneumolabyrinth should raise suspicion of a fistula.*

Post-traumatic Ossicular Chain Disruption

- Incudostapedial injury (subluxation or dislocation) is the most common trauma-related injury of the ossicles (Fig. 10), but often difficult to diagnose in the acute setting with haemotympanum often obscuring the joint.
- Incudostapedial joint is best seen on oblique reformations perpendicular to the oval window (refer Sect. 1 in chapter "Temporal Bone Imaging Techniques: Computer Tomography, Cone Beam CT and Magnetic Resonance Imaging").
- Malleoincudal subluxations may not be readily apparent on axial planes and hence needs to be evaluated on coronal planes as well (Fig. 11).
- The intact malleoincudal complex can be displaced en bloc, usually into the meso-tympanum (Fig. 12).
- If the incudostapedial and the malleoincudal joints are disrupted; then, the incus is said to be totally dislocated.
- Stapediovestibular dislocations and ossicular fractures are very rare.

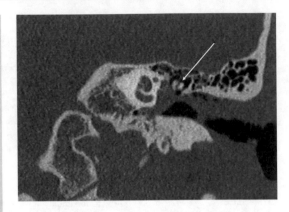

Fig. 11 Coronal CT in a post-traumatic patient (note the haemotympanum and blood in the EAC) shows widening of malleoincudal joint ("broken heart sign")

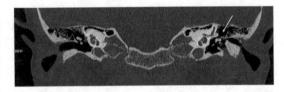

Fig. 12 Coronal CT image showing the malleoincudal complex being displaced inferiorly (arrow) from the epitympanum into the mesotympanum. Note the normal contralateral side for comparison

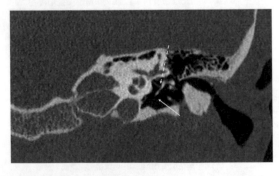

Fig. 10 Coronal CT image of a patient presenting with post-traumatic (note the deformity of the EAC) conductive hearing loss. There is complete dislocation of the incudostapedial joint with lentiform process of the incus (arrow) failing to articulate with the stapes head (dashed arrow), which accounts for the patient's symptoms

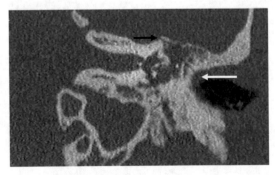

Fig. 13 Coronal CT image of a patient with post-traumatic otorrhea shows a tegmen fracture (black arrow) related to a longitudinal fracture traversing through the EAC (white arrow)

5   What the Surgeon Wants to Know (Table 5)

Table 5 Important checklist for reporting temporal bone trauma

What the surgeon wants to know	
Descriptor	Remember
Location and direction of fracture	• Use mixed classification, be aware of pseudo-fractures
Otic capsule violation	• Look for indirect signs like pneumolabyrinth
Ossicular integrity	• Compare with normal side for ossicular alignment • Use oblique reformations to visualize the joints and individual ossicles better • Dislocations are more common than ossicular fractures • Incudostapedial dislocation commonest followed by malleo-incudal
Facial nerve canal (does the facial nerve need to be decompressed?)	• Look for fracture line running close to the facial canal or subtle enlargement of geniculate fossa; if in doubt and clinical symptoms persist, suggest MRI • In acute palsy, a bony fracture fragment indenting on the nerve or loss of the normal canal borders is suspicious for impingement. • Facial nerve canal fracture can occur without any nerve dysfunction or overt impingement of the nerve
Tegmen: tympani and mastoideum	• Do not miss → short-term (meningitis, CSF leak) and long-term complications (encephalocele)
Vascular: carotid canal (petrous, cavernous), venous sinus (transverse, sigmoid and jugular bulb)	• ICA → dissection, occlusion, pseudoaneurysm or carotid-cavernous fistula • Traumatic venous sinus thrombosis • Suggest CT angio/venography when in doubt

Suggested Reading

Juliano AF, Ginat DT, Moonis G (2015) Imaging review of the temporal bone: part II. Traumatic, postoperative, and noninflammatory nonneoplastic conditions. Radiology 276:655–672

Kennedy TA, Avey GD, Gentry LR (2014) Imaging of temporal bone trauma. Neuroimaging Clin 24:467–486

Kwong Y, Yu D, Shah J (2012) Fracture mimics on temporal bone CT: a guide for the radiologist. AJR Am J Roentgenol 199(2):428–434. https://doi.org/10.2214/AJR.11.8012

Patel A, Groppo E (2010) Management of temporal bone trauma. Craniomaxillofac Trauma Reconstr 3: 105–113

Imaging of the Petrous Apex, Cerebellopontine Angles and Jugular Foramen

Dinesh Singh

Contents

Abstract

The petrous apex, cerebellopontine angles and jugular foramen have many important neurovascular structures traversing in and around them. The lesions in these areas are unfortunately varied and tend to overlap considerably. This chapter provides a concise overview of the relevant anatomy and a systematic stepwise approach on how to differentiate these various lesions.

D. Singh (✉)
Department of Diagnostic Radiology, Khoo Teck
Puat Hospital, Singapore, Singapore
e-mail: rambachan.singh.dinesh@ktph.com.sg

1 Petrous Apex

1.1 What Is the Petrous Apex and What Pathologies Involve It?

The petrous apex is the medially oriented pyramidal-shaped segment of the temporal bone that is surrounded by many important neurovascular structures (Fig. 1).

The associated pathologies can be broadly classified into *developmental, inflammatory, neoplastic and vascular* conditions. Variable degree of pneumatization (Fig. 1) and fatty marrow content can often result in "pseudo-lesions".

It is important to note that certain conditions can only arise if there is pre-existing pneumatization of the petrous apex, e.g. petrous apicitis, cholesterol granuloma, cholesteatoma and mucocele.

Petrous apex pathologies are often asymptomatic or present with non-specific symptoms such as headache or pain around the eye or ear. There may be associated cranial nerve neuropathy, with the trigeminal and abducens nerves being the commonest. Clinical diagnosis is often difficult; hence, imaging plays a key role in evaluation.

1.2 Choice of Imaging

MR imaging is the preferred imaging modality due to its excellent soft-tissue contrast, with many conditions being diagnosed just based on their characteristic MR appearance.

Non-contrast high-resolution CT of temporal bone is useful to look for any specific bony disease and to assess the pneumatization and matrix mineralization patterns, if needed.

1.3 Common Petrous Apex Lesions and its Differentials

Most petrous apex lesions have typical imaging features that make them easily recognizable; nonetheless, the below flow chart will simplify the differentiating process (Fig. 2).

The key imaging features of some of the common petrous apex lesions are summarized subsequently (Table 1).

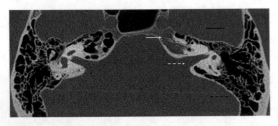

Fig. 1 Axial CT image showing the asymmetrical pneumatization of the petrous apices, more on the right. The petrous apex lies between the middle (black arrow) and posterior (black dashed arrow) cranial fossae, bounded by the petro-clival fissure medially (white arrow) and the inner ear structures laterally. The IAC (white dashed arrow) divides the petrous apex into larger anterior segment and a smaller posterior segment

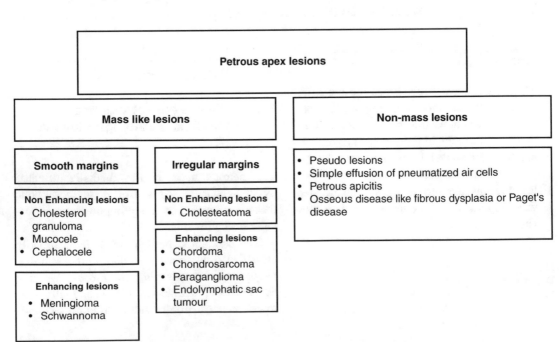

Fig. 2 Approach to petous apex pathologies

> **Tip**
> - *Asymmetric pneumatization of the petrous apex can give false impression of a lesion, especially on MR imaging; always double-check on CT if in doubt.*
> - *Imaging tends to be diagnostic in petrous apex lesions; if not then at least classify the lesion as benign or aggressive and delineate the extent.*

Table 1 Salient features of petrous apex lesions

Diagnosis	Key imaging findings	Remember
Cholesterol granuloma	• CT → expansile lesion associated with smooth bony remodelling • MRI → *Characteristic high signal on T1 and T2* (Fig. 3) with no restricted diffusion or enhancement	• Use fat-suppressed sequences to differentiate it from asymmetric bone marrow which may be bright on T1 as well
Mucocele	• CT → Expansile hypodense lesion with smooth scalloped borders • MRI → T1 iso or low signal with high T2 signal and no contrast enhancement	• Can mimic effusion • The low T1 signal differentiating it from Cholesterol granuloma
Cephalocele	• CT → Cystic lesion usually continuous with the Meckel cave, having smooth scalloped borders • MRI → *Signal mirrors that of CSF on all sequences*	• Usually incidental but hearing loss and CSF otorrhea are possible • Look for extension into the inner ear and signs of intracranial hypertension
Meningioma	• Dural-based lesion arising from the medial portion of the petrous apex (ptero-clival) or CPA • CT → Dense lesion with underlying hyperostosis and possible intralesional calcifications • MRI → Low to iso on T1W, iso to high on T2W images with avid post-contrast enhancement	• Broad base and dural tail usually differentiate it from other enhancing lesions like Schwannomas
Schwannoma	• Well-circumscribed enhancing mass • Can arise from trigeminal, facial or vestibulo-cochlear nerves • CT → Iso-dense • MRI → Low on T1 and high on T2-weighted images	• Larger lesions can show cystic changes and fluid-fluid levels • No dural tail or hyperostosis
Cholesteatoma	• CT → Expansile lesion with bony destruction • MRI → Iso to low on T1, high on T2W and *restricted diffusion on DWI*, non-enhancing	• Restricted diffusion on DWI is key
Chordoma/ chondrosarcoma	• CT → Expansile soft tissue mass with internal calcifications and surrounding bony erosions • MRI → Heterogenous low onT1 and high on T2 (can be higher than CSF signal) with variable enhancement (may show "honey-comb" pattern) • Chordoma tends to be a midline lesion centred on clivus (Fig. 4) • Chondrosarcoma tends to be more off midline, with widening of the petroclival fissure (Fig. 5)	• Benign vs malignant impossible to distinguish on imaging • "Ring and Arc" calcifications if present are characteristic • Associated with Maffucci syndrome, Ollier or Paget disease

(continued)

Table 1 (continued)

Diagnosis	Key imaging findings	Remember
Endolymphatic sac tumour	• CT → Soft tissue lesion with permeative bone destruction may show internal calcification (Fig. 6) and thin shell-like rim of overlying cortex • MRI → Variable heterogeneous signal on T1, T2 • MRI → May show flow voids and often demonstrate intense nodular enhancement • Some evidence of intra-lesional haemorrhage is usually seen	• Erosions classically along the posterior margin of the temporal bone • Bilateral tumour associated with von Hippel-Lindau disease (vHL)
Paraganglioma	• CT → Characteristic permeative bone destruction arising from the adjacent jugular foramen or middle ear, with intense contrast enhancement • Refer to Table 5	• Needs to be differentiated from other destructive lesions • Refer to Table 5
Petrous apicitis	• CT → Opacification of the pneumatized apical cells, mastoid air cells and middle ear cavity; bone erosions in late stages (Fig. 7) • MRI → Low on T1, high on T2 and post-contrast enhancement • Adjacent dural or cranial nerve enhancement	• Clinical presentation, Gradenigo' s triad • Look for abscess formation (Fig. 8), adjacent leptomeningeal enhancement (meningitis/encephalitis) and venous sinus thrombosis
Osseous disease	• Fibrous dysplasia can involve the petrous apex and shows typical "ground glass matrix" on CT, with bony expansion • Paget disease: lytic areas on CT in the early phase and bone thickening and sclerosis, in late stage	• CT is usually diagnostic (Fig. 9) • On MRI it can mimic tumour, look for general preservation of the petrous apex shape despite expansion and the intact hypointense line of the cortex

What the Surgeon Wants to Know?
• The relationship of the lesion with the petrous carotid artery; is it involved, spared and how far away is it?
• How does the lesion relate to the IAC and inner ear structures?
• Is the lesion accessible via the sphenoid sinus? (especially for cholesterol granuloma, mucocele and cholesteatoma)
  – Does the lesion lie in close proximity to the sphenoid sinus?
  – Is the sinus well aerated?
  – Does the internal carotid artery interpose between the sinus and the lesion?

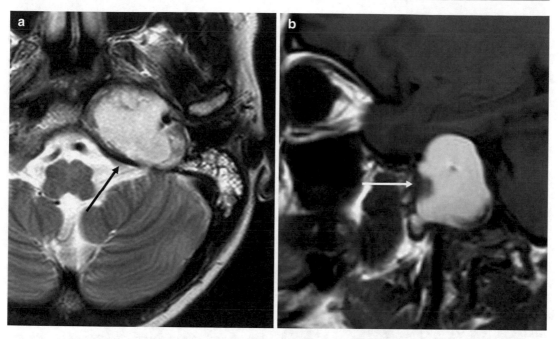

Fig. 3 (**a** and **b**) Axial T2 (**a**) and sagittal T1 MR (**b**) images show a hyperintense expansile petrous apex lesion showing signal characteristics typical for cholesterol granuloma (arrows)

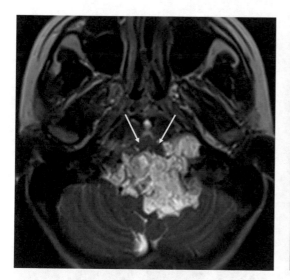

Fig. 4 Axial T2 MR image shows a hyperintense destructive lesion centred upon the clivus (arrows), consistent with Chordoma

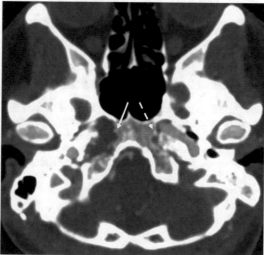

Fig. 5 Post contrast-enhanced axial CT image shows a destructive lesion centred on the right petrous apex with widening of the right petro-clival fissure (arrow), consistent with chondrosarcoma. The normal left petro-clival fissure is shown for comparison (dashed arrow)

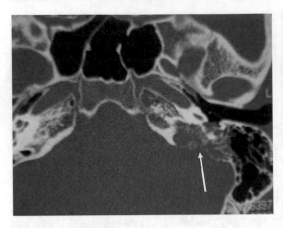

Fig. 6 Axial CT image shows a destructive lesion with faint internal calcifications and erosive changes along the posterior margin of the temporal bone (epicentre at the region of the endolymphatic sac), classical appearance of an endolymphatic sac tumour

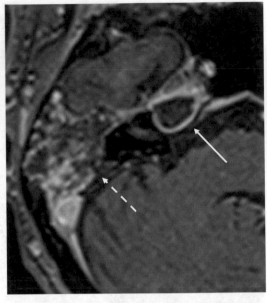

Fig. 8 Post-contrast axial MR image shows a ring-enhancing collection in the right petrous apex (white arrow) and mastoiditis (white dashed arrow). Also note the faint enhancement in the IAC indicating facial nerve involvement

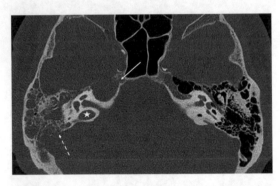

Fig. 7 CT axial image shows evidence of mastoiditis (white dashed arrow) and opacification of the right petrous apex (white arrow), note the destruction/erosion of the cortex around the pneumatized petrous apex. For comparison note the pneumatized and well-aerated left petrous apex and mastoid air cells. Incidental note is made of a high riding right jugular bulb (white star)

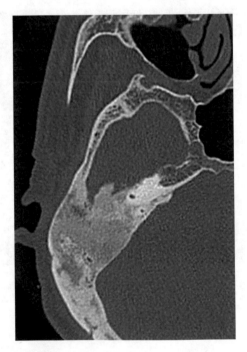

Fig. 9 Axial CT image shows ground-glass expansion of the temporal bone consistent with fibrous dysplasia

2   Cerebellopontine Angle

2.1   What Is the Cerebellopontine Angle and What Lesions Involve It?

The cerebellopontine angle (CPA) is an infratentorial subarachnoid space lateral to the pons, ventral to the cerebellum, limited anteriorly by the posterior margin of the petrous temporal bone and traversed by many important neurovascular structures.

The most common lesions of the CPA are the vestibular (cochlear nerve schwannoma is less common) schwannomas, followed by, meningiomas, arachnoid and epidermoid cysts.

Less common pathologies include other cranial nerve schwannomas (V, VII etc.), dermoid cysts, lipomas, metastases, vascular tumours, skull base and intra-axial tumours. Petrous apex pathologies can sometimes extend to involve the CPA.

The presentation depends largely on the size of the lesion and the degree of compression on the cranial nerves or brainstem (from cranial nerve palsy or hydrocephalus).

2.2   Choice of Imaging

Contrast-enhanced MRI is the imaging modality of choice for detection and delineation of tumour extent. CT of the temporal bone can depict the bony involvement if present (e.g. widening of the porus acousticus, erosions etc.), but demonstration of crucial neurovascular involvement is suboptimal.

2.3   Common Cerebellopontine Angle Lesions and its Differentials

As stated earlier, the potential lesions involving the CPA are vast. To narrow down the differentials, it is useful to divide the lesions as per their location (skull base, intra- and extra-axial lesions) and then its enhancement patterns (enhancing and non-enhancing) (Fig. 10).

The skull base lesions overlap with petrous apex lesions and have been enumerated earlier. Detailed description of intra-axial lesions is beyond the scope of this book. Key imaging features of some of the common extra-axial CPA lesions are summarized subsequently (Table 2).

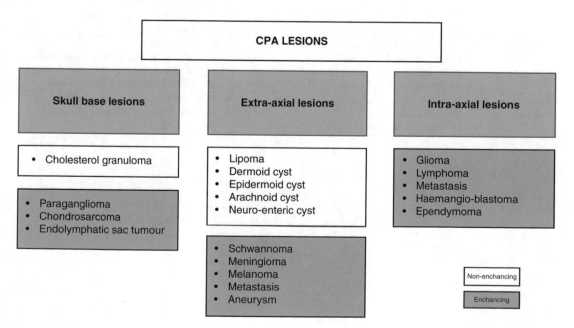

Fig. 10 CPA lesions

> **Tip**
> - *Vestibular Schwannomas are the most common CP angle tumour (80–85%) followed by meningioma. Bilateral CP angle lesions are suggestive of neurofibromatosis 2.*

Table 2 Cerebellopontine angle lesions

Diagnosis	Key imaging findings	Remember
Vestibular schwannoma	• "Ice cream cone" appearance (Fig. 11); canalicular (cone) and the cisternal (scoop) segments • CT → Typically iso-dense lesions (easily missed) • MRI → Same as Table 1	• Look for subtle asymmetric widening of the porus acousticus or scalloping along the IAC or CP angles on CT • Look for extension of the lesion into the cochlea or vestibule • Measure the "fundal fluid cap"
Meningioma	• CT and MRI. Same as Table 1	• Location is key, usually along the posterior aspect of the temporal bone or around the porus acousticus (Fig. 12) • The surface could be serrated and if it extends into the internal auditory canal (IAC), it usually does not widen the canal
Arachnoid cyst	• CT → Hypodense lesion with asymmetric enlargement of the CPA cistern • MRI → CSF signal on all sequences, no enhancement • Internal septa are better visualized on MRI	• DWI and FLAIR are useful for differentiation from epidermoid cyst
Epidermoid cyst	• CT → Hypodense lesions that conform to the shape of the CPA cistern • MRI → T1 and T2 similar to CSF, no over enhancement	• DWI → restricted diffusion (Fig. 13) • FLAIR → differs from CSF signal by being more heterogenous and hyperintense
Dermoid cyst	• CT → Mixed density lesion containing fat, calcification and soft tissue • MRI → Well-demarcated lesion with heterogeneous signal intensity, no enhancement	• Usually midline • A ruptured dermoid cyst can result in T1 high signal foci in the subarachnoid space or fat-fluid level within the ventricles
Vascular lesions	• Dolichoectasia, aneurysm or arterio-venous malformation (Fig. 14) • Diagnosis confirmed on CT/MR angiography	• Potential for neurovascular conflict • Aneurysm may mimic schwannoma on post-contrast images

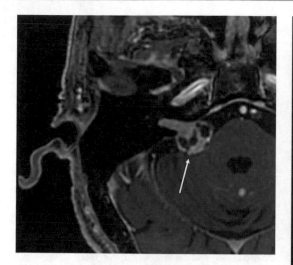

Fig. 11 Axial post-contrast MR image shows an avidly enhancing CPA lesion in "ice-cream cone" configuration showing a few non-enhancing cystic spaces (arrow) and indenting upon the middle cerebellar peduncle, consistent with a vestibular Schwannoma

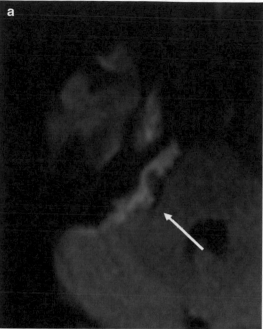

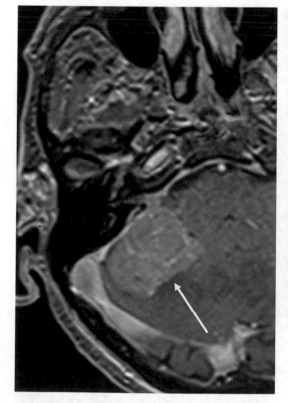

Fig. 12 Axial post-contrast MR image shows an enhancing broad-based lesion along the CPA (arrow) with dural enhancement extending into the IAM and exerting considerable mass effect on the cerebellum, consistent with meningioma

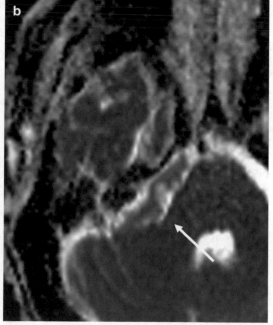

Fig. 13 (**a** and **b**) Axial DWI (**a**) and ADC (**b**) images show a CPA lesion with extension into the Meckel's cave depicting restricted diffusion, compatible with an epidermoid cyst

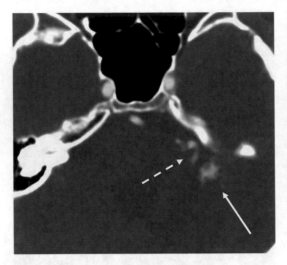

Fig. 14 Axial post-contrast CT image shows an arteriovenous malformation along the CPA (arrow) with a prominent draining vein (dashed arrow) medial to it

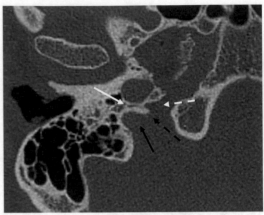

Fig. 15 Axial CT image shows the pars nervosa (white dashed arrow) and the pars vascularis (black arrow) separated by the jugular spine (black dashed arrow). The inferior tympanic canaliculus (white arrow) containing the Jacobsen's nerve arises from the pars nervosa

3 Jugular Foramen

3.1 What Constitutes the Jugular Foramen and What Pathologies Involve It?

The jugular foramen is a highly variable opening that lies between the petrous temporal bone laterally and the occipital bone medially (Figs. 15 and 16). The foramen is popularly (*but misleadingly*) divided into the smaller anteromedial "pars nervosa" and the posteromedial large "pars vascularis" by the jugular spine; both compartments transmit both vascular and neural components (Table 3).

Jugular foramen lesions can be classified into those primarily arising in this location, i.e. paragangliomas, schwannomas, meningiomas etc. and those arising from the adjacent structures that secondarily involve the foramen, e.g. chondrosarcomas and inflammatory lesions.

Remember
- **Jacobsen's nerve** is the tympanic branch of CN IX, and it lies within the

Table 3 Contents of the jugular foramen

Pars nervosa	Pars vascularis
Glossopharyngeal nerve (CN IX)	Vagus Nerve (CN X)
Jacobsen's nerve	Accessory nerve (CN XI)
Inferior petrosal sinus	Arnold's nerve
	Inferior jugular vein

inferior tympanic canaliculus (Fig. 15), which originates from the pars nervosa and extends to the tympanic cavity. Its clinical importance lies in the fact that it gives rise to the glomus tympanicum.
- **Arnold's nerve** is the mastoid branch of CN X, and it lies in the mastoid canaliculus (Fig. 16), which extends from the pars vascularis to the mastoid segment of the facial nerve. It is clinically important, since it can give rise to the glomus jugulo-tympanicum, represents a connection between the CN VII and CN X and can be the route for referred otalgia from the larynx.

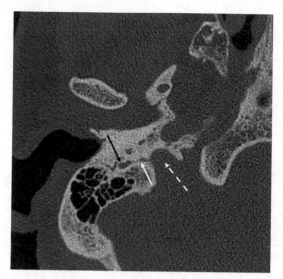

Fig. 16 Axial CT image shows the mastoid canaliculus (white arrow) containing Arnold's nerve arising from the pars vascularis (dashed white arrow) running towards the mastoid segment of the facial nerve (black arrow)

Jugular foramen lesions can present in a myriad of ways from simple headache to pulsatile tinnitus, but features of lower cranial nerve palsies, such as hoarseness, loss of taste, dysphagia or neck muscle weakness can be quite specific. Paragangliomas may present with unique symptoms such as headache, palpitations, nausea and sweating related to catecholamine surplus.

3.2 Choice of Imaging

Given the complexity of the jugular fossa foramen, CT and MR imaging are complementary. A high-resolution CT of the skull base is excellent in depicting the skull base anatomy and evaluating the pattern of bony changes (aggressive vs non-aggressive). CT angiography is useful in differentiating between paragangliomas and schwannomas, based on the degree of enhancement on arterial and venous phases. MR imaging has excellent soft tissue contrast and spatial resolution which enables detection of small lesions and delineating disease extent.

3.3 Intrinsic Jugular Foramen Lesions and Variants

Before tackling the actual lesions of the jugular foramen, it is vital to be aware of a few common anatomical variants that are encountered in this region (Table 4).

Table 4 Anatomical variants of the jugular bulb

Variant	Key imaging findings
Asymmetric enlargement of the jugular bulb	A dominant jugular bulb is usually noted, resulting in an ipsilateral enlarged jugular foramen with smooth rounded margins. Cortex remains intact and the jugular spine is preserved (pathology will invariably erode the jugular spine)
High-riding jugular bulb	Dome of the jugular bulb lies above the level of the inferior tympanic annulus or above the floor of the internal acoustic meatus – important pre-surgical finding (Fig.17)
Jugular bulb dehiscence	Protrusion of the jugular bulb or IJV into the middle ear cavity due to sigmoid plate dehiscence can be a cause of tinnitus

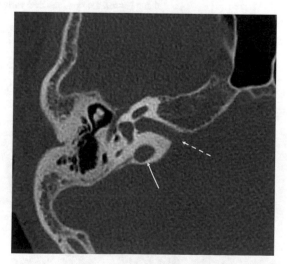

Fig. 17 Axial CT image shows a high riding jugular bulb (arrow) above the level of the IAC floor (dashed arrow)

Again, there is considerable overlap with the lesions encountered elsewhere in this chapter. The most important intrinsic lesion in this region is the glomus jugulare, and its key imaging features and that of some other common intrinsic lesions are described below (Table 5).

Table 5 Intrinsic jugular foramen lesions

Diagnosis	Key imaging findings	Important points
Glomus jugulare paraganglioma	• Permeative bone destruction around the jugular foramen (best on CT) (Fig. 18) • The tumour often invades the jugular bulb, the sigmoid sinus and extends to the carotid space and mastoid air cells • The tumour may extend through the jugular plate into the middle ear, destroying the ossicles (glomus jugulo-tympanicum) • MRI → Classically "salt and pepper" appearance on T1 images in tumours greater than 2 cm in size (Fig. 19) • "Pepper" represents the low signal from high-velocity vascular flow voids • "Salt" is the high signal due to focal subacute haemorrhages • Marked enhancement, which is brighter than T2 fluid and shows rapid wash-out	• Up to 80% of jugular foramen tumours • "Salt and pepper" appearance is diagnostic but only obvious in larger lesions • Catheter angiogram is useful for providing a vascular road map and pre-operative embolization by identifying the feeding arteries (most commonly from the ascending pharyngeal artery) • Associations: MEN 2, NF 1, Von Hippel-Lindau syndrome
Schwannoma	• Similar imaging appearance to lesions in the petrous apex and CPA • CT → soft tissue mass enlarging the jugular fossa, iso-dense to the brain parenchyma, smooth margins and causing bony scalloping and erosion of the jugular spine • MRI → low T1, high T2 signal intensity mass with prominent enhancement • Larger lesions can demonstrate degenerative changes with cystic areas and variable enhancement	• Tumours follow the course of the lower cranial nerves • Ninth nerve schwannoma usually grows in supero-medial direction, towards the brainstem (Fig. 20) • 10th and 11th nerve schwannomas typically grow inferiorly towards the neck
Primary jugular fossa meningioma	• Usually en-plaque lesion with enhancing dural tail • CT and MRI → Same as Table 1	• Same as Table 1

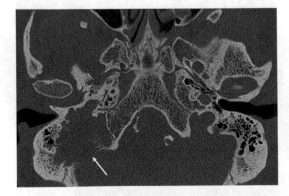

Fig. 18 Axial CT image shows a permeative destructive lesion centred on the right jugular foramen (arrow), the contralateral normal side is given for comparison

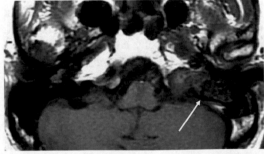

Fig. 19 Axial T1 MR image shows a glomus jugulare lesion in the left temporal bone with numerous hypointense flow voids interspersed with few hyperintense foci giving rise to the classical "salt and pepper" appearance

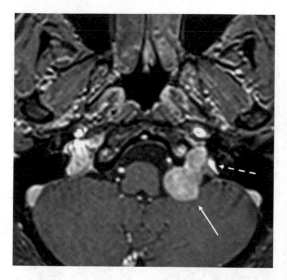

Fig. 20 Axial contrast-enhanced MRI shows a well-demarcated enhancing lesion (arrow) arising from an enlarged pars nervosa compatible with a glossopharyngeal Schwannoma. The non-dominant IJV is seen adjacent to it (dashed arrow)

Tip
- *Sometimes a large glomus jugulare lesion can extend to the tympanic cavity, and the origin of the lesion is difficult to discern, i.e. is this a large glomus tympanicum or jugulare lesion; in such case use the term glomus jugulotympanicum*
- *IJV thrombophlebitis with its enhancing walls and perivascular oedema could potentially mimic a lesion.*

ELTS Vs. Glomus Jugulare

ELST, if large and involving the jugular foramen, can be mistaken for glomus jugulare, as these two lesions share some similar imaging features, such as destructive bony changes on CT scan, subacute haemorrhage and vascularity giving it a potential "salt and pepper" appearance on MR T1W sequences as well as intense post-gadolinium enhancement (Fig. 21). However, there are certain imaging features that could help differentiate ELST from glomus jugulare:

- As the name suggests, the epicentre of ELST is the endolymphatic sac, whereas glomus jugulare is centred upon the jugular foramen
- In glomus jugulare, the jugular spine is invariably destroyed, whereas in ELST, the jugular spine might still be preserved (Fig. 22).
- As mentioned earlier, in ELST intralesional calcifications/bony spicules are characteristic

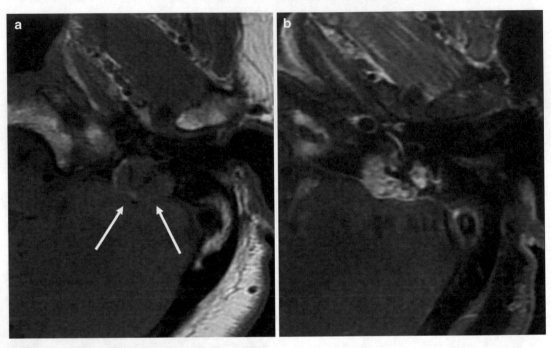

Fig. 21 (**a** and **b**) Axial T1W image (**a**) of the left middle ear cleft shows a heterogeneous lesion (arrows) with hypo and hyperintense internal foci representing vascular flow voids and subacute haemorrhage respectively. Post-contrast-enhanced axial image (**b**) shows this lesion to be intensely enhancing

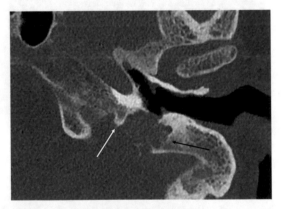

Fig. 22 Axial CT image shows destructive lesion with internal bony spicules (black arrow) involving the jugular foramen but with preservation of the jugular spine (white arrow). Findings are consistent with an endolymphatic sac tumour

Further Reading

Bonneville F, Savatovsky J, Chiras J (2007) Imaging of cerebellopontine angle lesions: an update. Part 1: enhancing extra-axial lesions. Eur Radiol 17(10):2472–2482

Bonneville F, Savatovsky J, Chiras J (2007) Imaging of cerebellopontine angle lesions: an update. Part 2: intra-axial lesions, skull base lesions that may invade the CPA region, and non-enhancing extra-axial lesions. Eur Radiol 17(11):2908–2920

Razek AA, Huang BY (2012) Lesions of the petrous apex: classification and findings at CT and MR imaging. Radiographics 32(1):151–173

Vogl TJ, Bisdas S (2009) Differential diagnosis of jugular foramen lesions. Skull Base 19(1):3–16

Imaging of the Facial Nerve: Approach and Pathology

Vishal Pralhad Gaikwad and Tiong Yong Tan

Contents

Abstract

The facial nerve is often impaired, and its evaluation can be complex. This chapter provides an insight into the relevant anatomy, suggestions for localizing lesions based on symptoms and guidelines on how to image the nerve adequately. The potential causes of facial nerve palsy and its differentials are discussed in an intuitive manner.

V. P. Gaikwad
Department of Diagnostic Radiology, Tan Tock Seng
Hospital, Singapore, Singapore
e-mail: vishal.gaikwad@mohh.com.sg

T. Y. Tan (✉)
Department of Radiology, Changi General Hospital,
Singapore, Singapore
e-mail: tan.tiong.yong@singhealth.com.sg

1 Facial Nerve Segments

The facial nerve contains motor, sensory and parasympathetic fibres and is the most commonly paralyzed nerve; as such imaging plays an important role in evaluating it. Given the scope of this book, only segments pertaining to the temporal bone are discussed (Table 1) (refer chapter "Basic Temporal Bone Imaging Anatomy: External, Middle and Inner Ear" for more details).

2 Imaging of the Facial Nerve

MRI is the imaging modality of choice with CT of the temporal bone being complimentary whenever bone disease is suspected or surgery is contemplated. Generally, contrast-enhanced MR is used to evaluate cisternal, intracanalicular segment or brainstem nuclei, while the labyrinthine,

Table 1 Facial nerve imaging pearls

Segment	Description	Branches	Remember
Cisternal	From pons to IAC, runs anterior to CN VIII	No branches	• Look for neurovascular conflict
Intra-canalicular	Segment within the IAC lies in the antero-superior quadrant	No branches	• Enhancing lesions in the IAC are more likely to be vestibular Schwannoma rather than facial nerve (unless very small and you can localize it to the CN VII)
Labyrinthine	From entry into the fallopian canal till geniculate ganglion	Greater superficial petrosal nerve (GSPN), lesser petrosal and external petrosal nerves	• Shortest and narrowest segment • Frequently involved in temporal bone fractures
Tympanic	From geniculate ganglion to posterior genu of facial nerve	No Branches	• Look for dehiscence, especially in cases of cholesteatoma
Mastoid	From posterior genu to stylomastoid mastoid foramen, vertical course behind the EAC	Nerve to stapedius and Chorda tympani	• Look for involvement in coalescent mastoiditis and destructive lesion around the EAC or jugular foramen
Extra-cranial	Beyond the stylomastoid foramen into the parotid space	Five terminal branches – temporal, zygomatic, buccal, mandibular and cervical	• The facial nerve divides the parotid gland into superficial and deep parts • Look for parotid malignancy and perineural spread

Table 2 Symptom based localization of facial nerve lesions

Symptomatology	Localization
Contralateral paresis of lower face with forehead sparing	Supranuclear lesion
Paresis/paralysis of ipsilateral forehead and lower face	Nuclear lesion
Loss of all three special senses is present along with abducens nerve palsy	Most likely at the level of lower pontine nuclei
Only deficiency of lacrimation	At the level of GSPN
Stapedius reflex dysfunction	Mastoid segment (near facial recess)
Loss of sensation of anterior two-third tongue	Level of lingual nerve (mastoid segment)
If all three special sensations are preserved with the presence of asymmetric loss of facial expression	Along extracranial segment

tympanic and mastoid segments can be evaluated by both CT and contrast-enhanced MR.

MR of facial nerve should have pre- and post-gadolinium axial and coronal T1W (3 mm with 10% inter-slice gap and small FOV) images and axial three-dimensional constructive interference in steady state-3D CISS (0.7 mm section). CT temporal bone should have 0.8-mm-thick slices acquired in an axial plane with coronal reformats. Axial plane is parallel to lateral semi-circular canal. Coronal oblique plane is perpendicular to the lateral semi-circular canal.

3   Localization of Facial Nerve Lesions (Topognosis)

A thorough neurological examination and history taking will allow for fairly accurate localization of any potential lesion along the various segments of the nerve (Table 2).

4 Facial Nerve Palsy

The potential causes for facial nerve palsy are extremely varied, but the most common cause remains inflammation or infection, followed by traumatic injury and neoplasm.

4.1 Inflammation

Bell's palsy contributes to the majority of cases under this particular cause. Typical Bell's palsy is a clinical diagnosis and usually does not require radiological evaluation unless the presentation is atypical, i.e. recurrent or sub-acute onset, progressive or prolonged palsy persisting for more than 4 months and multiple cranial nerve involvement.

Classical MR finding is that of uniform intra-temporal facial nerve enhancement without nerve enlargement or nodularity. The enhancement pattern is such that those portions of the facial nerve that usually enhance physiologically, like the geniculate ganglion, tympanic and mastoid segments, will enhance more intensely in Bell's palsy, and those that usually do not enhance, like the cisternal (IAC portion) and labyrinthine segments, will enhance pathologically (Fig. 1).

Ramsay Hunt Syndrome (shingles of the facial nerve) classically presents with painful vesicular

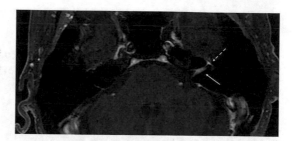

Fig. 2 Axial post-contrast MR image of a patient with Ramsay Hunt syndrome shows avid smooth enhancement in the IAC (arrow) involving the surrounding meninges, as well as abnormal enhancement along the labyrinthine and tympanic segments of the facial nerve (dashed arrow). Note the distinct lack of enhancement on the contralateral normal side

eruptions in and around the external auditory canal and facial nerve palsy (eighth nerve involvement can occur); it can be indistinguishable from Bell's palsy if no rash is present. MR findings are similar to Bell's palsy, but additionally the 8th nerve, the meninges within the IAC and membranous labyrinth can abnormally enhance as well (Fig. 2).

> **Remember**
> - Faint enhancement of geniculate ganglion, tympanic and mastoid segments is considered normal (in Bell's palsy these would enhance more intensely)
> - Enhancement of cisternal, intracanalicular, labyrinthine and extra-cranial segments of the facial nerve is always pathological
> - Even asymmetric thickening and enhancement of tympanic and mastoid segments is deemed abnormal

4.2 Injury/Trauma

Facial nerve injury common in temporal bone fractures and most often in transverse fractures. The nerve can be partially or completely transected, compressed or stretched with intra-neural oedema or hematoma. The most commonly

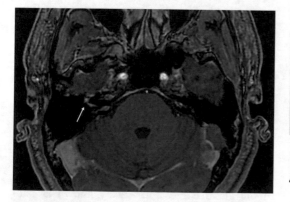

Fig. 1 Axial post-contrast MR image of a patient with Bell's palsy shows avid enhancement along the distal intra-canalicular and labyrinthine segments of the facial nerve as well as the geniculate ganglion (arrow). Note the distinct lack of enhancement on the contralateral normal side

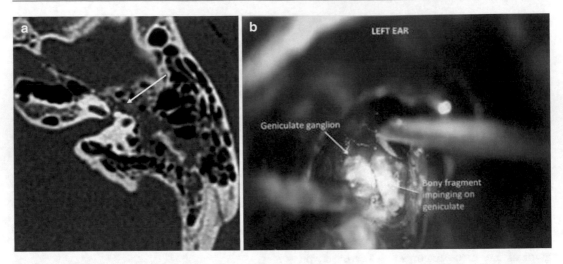

Fig. 3 (**a** and **b**) Axial CT image (**a**) of a temporal bone fracture shows loss of the lateral wall of the geniculate ganglion (arrow) with corresponding intra-operative image (**b**)

involved are the labyrinthine segment with transverse fractures and the geniculate ganglion with longitudinal fractures.

In post-traumatic facial nerve palsy of immediate onset, the main issue is whether there is impingement onto the facial nerve that requires surgical decompression. Determination of facial nerve impingement is, therefore, an important part of assessment in post-traumatic temporal bone scan. The mere presence of fracture line extending into the facial nerve canal does not equate to impingement. The sign for impingement is the disruption of the facial nerve canal margin by a bony fragment (Fig. 3).

> **Tip**
> • *In post-traumatic facial palsy without any obvious temporal bone fracture, the radiologist should assume that an occult temporal fracture is present. MRI studies in such scenarios can demonstrate abnormal facial nerve and dural enhancement along the temporal bone, probably due to micro-tears from micro-fractures.*

4.3 Neoplasms

Primary neoplasms of the facial nerve are rare with Schwannoma being the more common type and usually involves the geniculate ganglion (can involve more than one segment). Symptoms can be due to neural compression (palsy), pressure erosion of ossicles (CHL) or if cisternal or intracanalicular segments are involvement then sensorineural hearing loss could be present.

CT shows a well-defined lobulated mass causing fusiform enlargement of the facial nerve canal (Fig. 4). Bony changes (scalloping), if encountered, are due to chronic pressure rather than invasion and thus tend to be smooth and well defined. MRI is advantageous over CT due to its ability to appreciate the intense homogeneous enhancement (Fig. 5); lesions tend to be hyperintense on T2-weighted images and iso- to hypointense on T1-weighted images.

A possible differential for facial nerve Schwannoma is 'venous vascular malformation of the facial nerve' (previously known as haemangioma), which tends to be centred around the geniculate ganglion. The clinical presentation tends to be earlier, more severe and disproportionate to size of lesion compared to a Schwannoma, due to its invasive nature.

CT shows facial nerve enlargement with indistinct margins for non-ossifying type of haemangioma (in schwannoma, the margins are well defined). The ossifying variant may show classical spoke wheel or honey-comb appearance (Fig. 6). MR findings are unfortunately non-specific with heterogenous signal encountered on both T1- and T2-weighted images.

Tip
- *Always evaluate the parotid gland for possible malignancy in cases of idiopathic facial nerve palsy. Nearly half of parotid adenoid cystic carcinoma show perineural spread through the stylomastoid foramen (along the mastoid segment).*

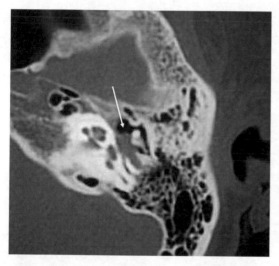

Fig. 4 CT axial image shows fusiform enlargement of the tympanic segment of the facial nerve (arrow). The lesion abuts the middle ear ossicles and shows intense post-contrast enhancement (not shown) compatible with a facial nerve Schwannoma

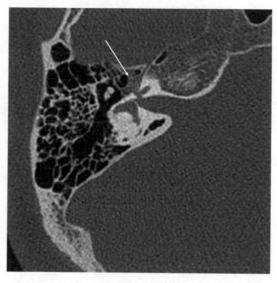

Fig. 6 Axial CT image shows an expansile lytic lesion with fine internal spiculations centred upon the geniculate ganglion of the facial nerve (arrow), classical appearance of an ossifying variant of a venous vascular malformation of the facial nerve. (Courtesy Dr. Julian Goh, Tan Tock Seng Hospital, Singapore)

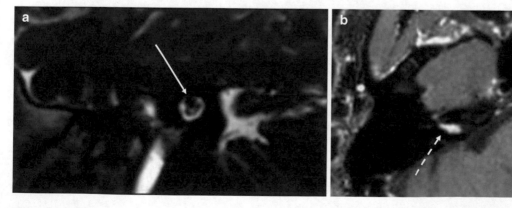

Fig. 5 (**a** and **b**) MR Sagittal T2 space sequence (**a**) shows a focal enlargement of the cisternal segment of the facial nerve in antero-superior quadrant of the IAM (arrow). Post-contrast axial T1 MR image (**b**) shows intense enhancement of the lesion, consistent with a Schwannoma (dashed arrow)

Further Reading

Chan EH, Tan HM, Tan TY (2005) Facial palsy from temporal bone lesions. Ann Acad Med Singap 34(4):322–329. Review

Haller S, Etienne L, Kövari E, Varoquaux AD, Urbach H, Becker M (2016) Imaging of neurovascular compression syndromes: trigeminal neuralgia, hemifacial spasm, vestibular paroxysmia, and glossopharyngeal neuralgia. AJNR Am J Neuroradiol 37(8):1384–1392. https://doi.org/10.3174/ajnr.A4683

Ho ML, Juliano A, Eisenberg RL, Moonis G (2015) Anatomy and pathology of the facial nerve. AJR Am J Roentgenol 204(6):W612–W619. https://doi.org/10.2214/AJR.14.13444

Mundada P, Purohit BS, Kumar TS, Tan TY (2016) Imaging of facial nerve schwannomas: diagnostic pearls and potential pitfalls. Diagn Interv Radiol 22(1):40–46. https://doi.org/10.5152/dir.2015.15060

Printed in the United States
by Baker & Taylor Publisher Services